The Complete Diabetic Cookbook for Beginners

2000 Days of Quick & Easy Low-Carb, Low-Sugar Diabetic Recipes with a 30-Day Meal Plan to Manage Type 2 Diabetes, Prediabetes and the Newly Diagnosed

Linette Johnston

Legal & Disclaimer

The information presented in this book has been compiled from reliable sources and reflects the author's best knowledge, expertise, and belief. While every effort has been made to ensure accuracy, the author assumes no responsibility for any errors or omissions.

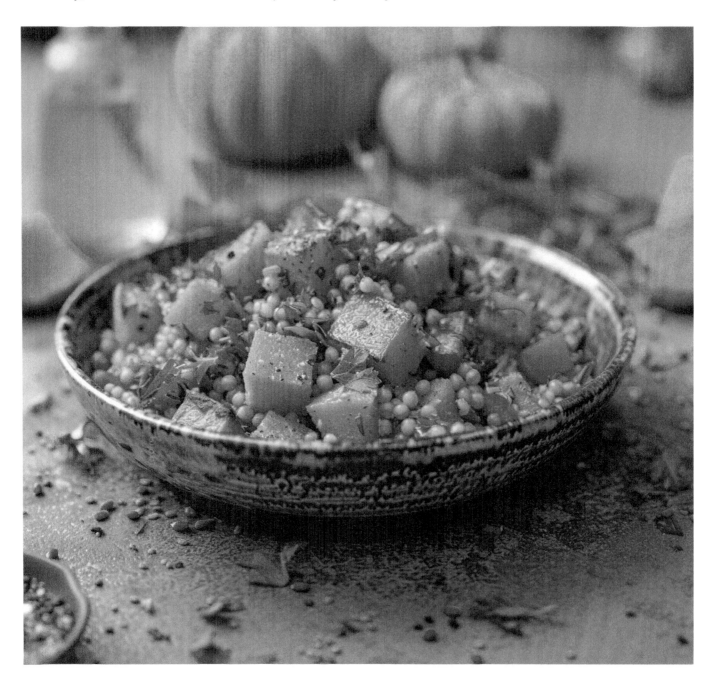

TABLE OF CONTENTS

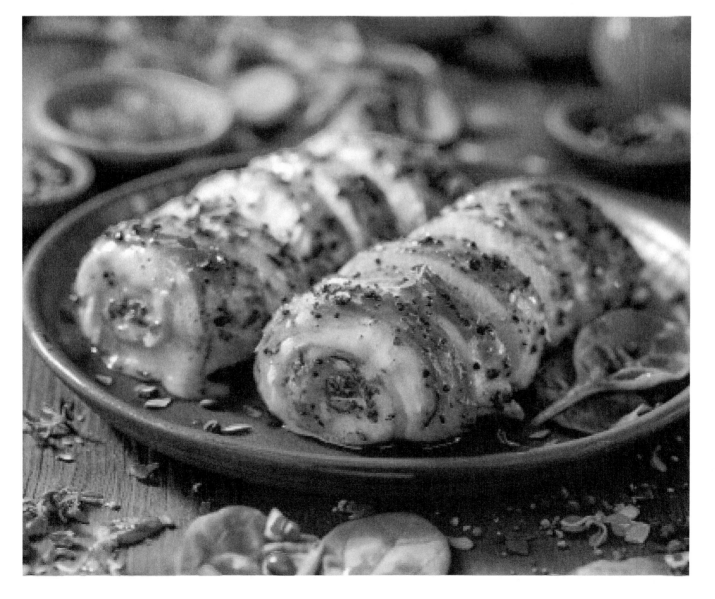

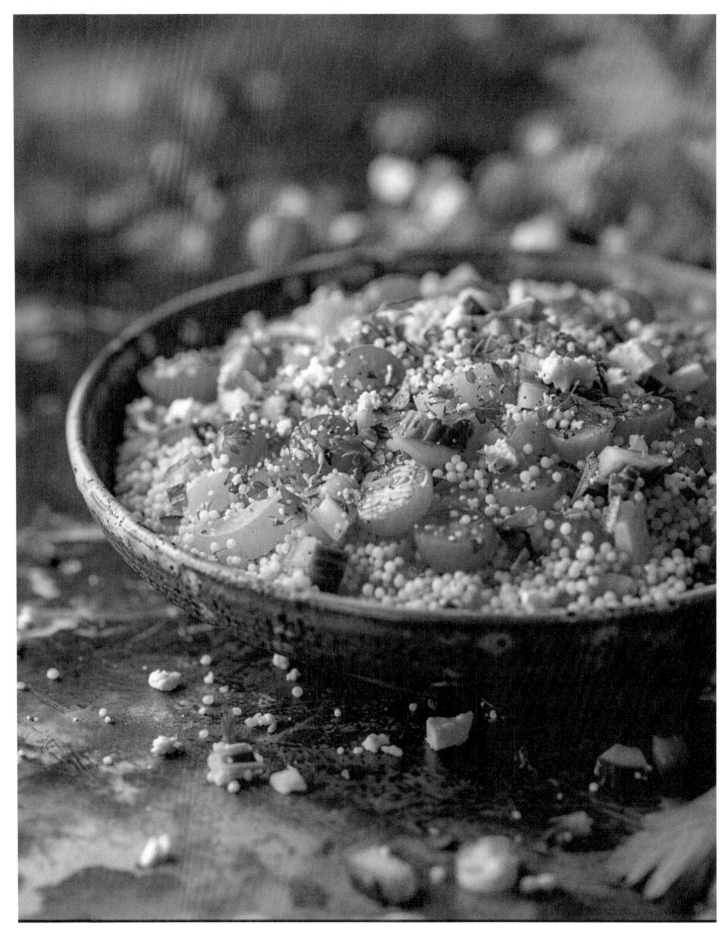

INTRODUCTION

Dear readers,

Linette Johnston is a celebrated professional chef and a distinguished expert in the realm of healthy eating, specializing in diabetic-friendly cuisine. Her unwavering passion for crafting meals that are both delicious and conducive to managing diabetes has established her as an authoritative figure in health-conscious cooking. With an in-depth understanding of nutrition and its impact on well-being, Linette merges culinary artistry with health science to create recipes that promote wellness without sacrificing flavor.

Her culinary creations are a symphony of tastes, colors, and textures, thoughtfully designed to delight the senses while supporting dietary needs. Linette firmly believes that adhering to a healthy diet doesn't mean compromising on enjoyment. This philosophy is evident throughout her work, where she emphasizes the balance between savoring food and maintaining optimal health.

Linette's journey into mastering diabetic-friendly cooking is both professional and deeply personal. She understands the complexities and challenges that come with embracing a new dietary lifestyle, especially for those newly diagnosed with diabetes. Her own transformative experiences inspire her mission to guide and support others on their path to wellness.

In her book, "The Complete Diabetic Cookbook for Beginners," Linette Johnston channels her expertise and passion to provide readers with invaluable tools and insights for achieving their health goals. She is dedicated to making the journey toward healthier living not just attainable but also enjoyable and rich in culinary delight. Her aim is to dispel the notion that diabetic diets are restrictive by showcasing recipes that are as exciting as they are nutritious.

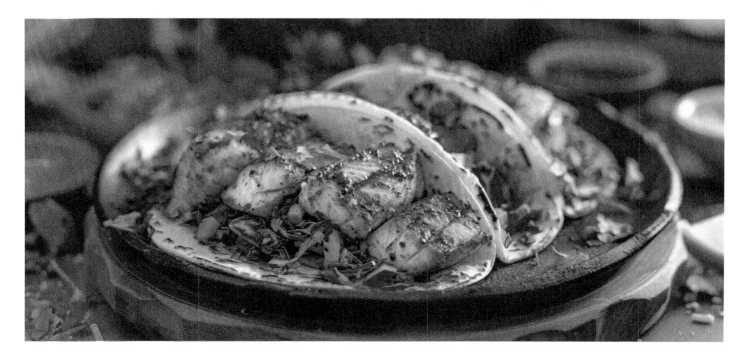

CHAPTER 1: THE FUNDAMENTALS OF DIABETES AND NUTRITION

Embarking on a journey with Type 2 diabetes or prediabetes can be challenging, but understanding how your diet impacts your blood sugar levels is a crucial first step toward effective management. I'm Linette Johnston, a professional chef dedicated to creating delicious, diabetes-friendly recipes. Together, we'll explore the relationship between food and diabetes and how to build a balanced, satisfying diet that supports your health goals.

What Is Diabetes?

Diabetes is a metabolic disorder characterized by high levels of glucose in the blood due to the body's inability to produce or effectively use insulin. When we eat, our bodies break down carbohydrates into glucose, which enters the bloodstream. Insulin, a hormone produced by the pancreas, helps cells absorb glucose to use for energy. In diabetes, this process is impaired—either the pancreas doesn't produce enough insulin, or the body's cells become resistant to it—leading to elevated blood sugar levels.

- **Type 2 Diabetes**: The most common form, where the body's cells become resistant to insulin.

- **Prediabetes**: A condition where blood sugar levels are higher than normal but not yet high enough for a diabetes diagnosis.

The encouraging news is that early intervention through diet and lifestyle changes can prevent or delay the progression from prediabetes to Type 2 diabetes.

Why Diet Is Key

Your diet plays a pivotal role in managing blood sugar levels. The foods you choose directly influence your glucose levels, making dietary choices essential for keeping diabetes under control. A diabetes-friendly diet focuses on balancing carbohydrates, proteins, and fats while prioritizing foods that minimize blood sugar spikes.

The Role of Carbohydrates

Carbohydrates have the most significant impact on blood sugar levels. However, not all carbs are created equal:

- **Complex Carbohydrates**: Found in whole grains, vegetables, and legumes. They are digested slowly, leading to gradual increases in blood sugar.

- **Simple Carbohydrates and Sugars**: Found in refined grains and sugary foods. They cause rapid spikes in blood sugar, which can be harder to control.

In this cookbook, I focus on selecting the right kinds of carbs in appropriate portions, helping you enjoy your meals without worrying about sudden glucose spikes.

Fats and Proteins: Your Allies

While carbohydrates are a major focus, healthy fats and proteins play essential roles in a diabetes-friendly diet.

- **Healthy Fats**: Found in olive oil, avocados, nuts, and fatty fish like salmon. They help you feel full and can slow the absorption of carbohydrates, preventing sharp increases in blood sugar.

- **Proteins**: Found in lean meats, poultry, fish, eggs, and plant-based sources like legumes and tofu. They help stabilize glucose levels and promote satiety.

My recipes thoughtfully incorporate these nutrients to enhance flavor while supporting blood sugar balance.

The Importance of Portion Control

Portion control is another critical aspect of managing diabetes. Even healthy foods can lead to high blood sugar if consumed in large amounts. Learning to gauge portions and understanding your body's unique response to certain foods is key to long-term success. Throughout this book, I provide practical portion guidelines, ensuring you can enjoy delicious meals while staying on track with your health goals.

Hydration and Blood Sugar

Staying hydrated is essential for everyone, but it's especially important when managing diabetes.

- **Water**: Helps regulate blood sugar levels and supports overall health.

- **Sugary Beverages**: Can lead to rapid blood sugar spikes and should be avoided.

This cookbook includes refreshing, low-sugar drink options to keep you hydrated without risking your glucose levels.

Mindful Eating for Lasting Results

Beyond what you eat, how you approach meals can make a significant difference.

- **Mindful Eating**: Involves taking the time to savor your food and listen to your body's hunger and fullness cues.

- **Benefits**: Helps you feel more satisfied, reduces overeating, and enhances your overall eating experience.

I encourage a balanced, mindful approach to eating, ensuring that meals are not just about nutrition but also about enjoyment and fulfillment.

Additional Insights: The Power of Fiber and Meal Timing

Embracing Fiber

Fiber is a type of carbohydrate that the body can't digest, and it offers numerous benefits:

- **Blood Sugar Control**: Slows the absorption of sugar, helping to improve blood sugar levels.

- **Heart Health**: Can lower cholesterol levels.

- **Sources**: Whole grains, legumes, vegetables, fruits, nuts, and seeds.

Timing Your Meals

Eating regular, balanced meals can prevent significant fluctuations in blood sugar levels.

- **Consistency**: Aim for consistent meal times.
- **Frequency**: Smaller, more frequent meals may help maintain steadier glucose levels.

Building a Supportive Lifestyle

Managing diabetes isn't solely about diet; it's part of a broader lifestyle approach that includes physical activity, regular medical check-ups, and stress management.

Physical Activity

- **Benefits**: Enhances insulin sensitivity and aids in blood sugar control.
- **Activities**: Walking, swimming, dancing, gardening—choose activities you enjoy to make it sustainable.

Stress Management

- **Impact**: Stress can affect blood sugar levels by releasing hormones like cortisol.
- **Techniques**: Deep breathing exercises, meditation, yoga, or engaging in hobbies.

Your Journey Ahead

Starting this journey may seem daunting, but every step you take is a move toward better health. This cookbook is designed to make that journey enjoyable and delicious. With over 2,000 days of carefully crafted recipes and a 30-day meal plan, you'll find inspiration and support to manage your diabetes effectively.

Let's begin this culinary adventure together, embracing foods that nourish your body and delight your palate.

The Science Behind the Diabetic Diet

Understanding the scientific principles behind the diabetic diet is essential for effectively managing Type 2 diabetes and prediabetes.

The Role of Blood Sugar and Insulin

At the core of diabetes management are two key players: blood sugar (glucose) and insulin. When you consume carbohydrates, your body breaks them down into glucose, which enters the bloodstream. In response, the pancreas releases insulin—a hormone that helps cells absorb glucose to use for energy.

In Type 2 diabetes, however, the body either doesn't produce enough insulin or becomes resistant to its effects. This insulin resistance leads to elevated blood sugar levels, which, if unmanaged, can result in serious health complications such as heart disease, nerve damage, and kidney issues.

How the Diabetic Diet Helps

A well-designed diabetic diet focuses on foods that minimize blood sugar spikes, improve insulin sensitivity, and promote overall metabolic health. By carefully selecting what you eat, you can help regulate glucose levels and reduce the risk of complications associated with diabetes.

The Glycemic Index: Choosing Carbohydrates Wisely

One fundamental concept is the Glycemic Index (GI), which ranks carbohydrates based on how quickly they raise blood sugar levels. Low-GI foods (like whole grains, legumes, and non-starchy vegetables) are digested slowly, leading to a gradual rise in blood sugar. High-GI foods (such as white bread, sugary snacks, and refined grains) cause rapid spikes.

By prioritizing low-GI carbohydrates, you can achieve more stable blood sugar levels. In this cookbook, I've crafted recipes that emphasize low-GI ingredients, allowing you to enjoy delicious meals without compromising your health.

The Power of Fiber

Fiber is a type of carbohydrate that the body can't digest, and it plays a crucial role in a diabetic-friendly diet. Found in fruits, vegetables, whole grains, and legumes, fiber slows down digestion and the absorption of sugars, leading to a more gradual rise in blood glucose after meals.

- **Benefits of Fiber**:
    - Improves blood sugar control
    - Enhances insulin sensitivity
    - Supports digestive health
    - Promotes a feeling of fullness, aiding in weight management

My recipes incorporate fiber-rich ingredients to help you harness these benefits while enjoying flavorful dishes.

Balancing Macronutrients for Optimal Health

While managing carbohydrates is essential, balancing your intake of proteins and fats is equally important.

Proteins: Building Blocks and Blood Sugar Stabilizers

Protein has a minimal effect on blood glucose levels and is vital for building and repairing tissues.

- **Lean Protein Sources**:
    - Poultry (chicken, turkey)
    - Fish (salmon, tuna)
    - Plant-based options (tofu, legumes)
    - Low-fat dairy products

Including adequate protein in your meals can help you feel satisfied and maintain steady blood sugar levels.

Healthy Fats: Supporting Heart Health

Not all fats are created equal. Healthy fats are essential for nutrient absorption and can improve heart health—a significant consideration for people with diabetes.

- **Sources of Healthy Fats**:
    - Monounsaturated fats (olive oil, avocados, nuts)
    - Omega-3 fatty acids (fatty fish like salmon, flaxseeds, walnuts)

Conversely, it's important to limit unhealthy fats such as trans fats and excessive saturated fats, which can increase the risk of heart disease.

The Importance of Portion Control and Meal Timing

Portion Control

Understanding appropriate portion sizes helps prevent overeating, which can lead to blood sugar imbalances and weight gain.

- **Tips for Portion Control**:

  - Use smaller plates to help control portions visually

  - Measure servings with measuring cups or a food scale

  - Be mindful of serving sizes listed on nutrition labels

Throughout this book, I've included portion guidelines to assist you in enjoying meals without overindulging.

Meal Timing

Eating regular, well-spaced meals can prevent significant fluctuations in blood sugar levels.

- **Benefits of Consistent Meal Timing**:

  - Maintains steady glucose levels

  - Reduces the risk of hypoglycemia (low blood sugar)

  - Helps manage hunger and prevent overeating

Consider planning your meals and snacks at consistent times each day to support optimal blood sugar control.

Why a Low-Carb Diet is Effective for Diabetes Management

Research has shown that a low-carbohydrate diet can significantly improve blood sugar control in individuals with diabetes. By reducing the intake of high-carb foods, especially refined sugars and starches, you can lower post-meal glucose spikes.

- **Benefits of a Low-Carb Diet**:

  - Improved glycemic control

  - Enhanced weight management

  - Increased insulin sensitivity

In **"The Complete Diabetic Cookbook for Beginners"**, the recipes are designed with these principles in mind, focusing on low-carb, nutrient-dense ingredients that make managing diabetes both effective and enjoyable.

The Value of Personalization

Every individual's experience with diabetes is unique. Factors such as age, activity level, medications, and personal preferences influence how your body responds to different foods.

- **Personalizing Your Diet**:

  - Monitor your blood sugar levels to see how different foods affect you

  - Work with a healthcare professional or dietitian to tailor your diet plan

  - Adjust recipes to suit your taste and nutritional needs

This cookbook offers a wide array of recipes and meal plans to accommodate diverse tastes and lifestyles, empowering you to take control of your health in a way that suits you best.

Additional Insights: Beyond Diet

While diet plays a pivotal role, incorporating other healthy habits enhances diabetes management.

Physical Activity

Regular exercise helps improve insulin sensitivity and aids in blood sugar control.

- **Types of Beneficial Activities**:
  - Aerobic exercises (walking, swimming, cycling)
  - Strength training (weightlifting, resistance bands)
  - Flexibility and balance exercises (yoga, tai chi)

Aim for at least 150 minutes of moderate-intensity aerobic activity per week, as recommended by health guidelines.

Stress Management

Chronic stress can negatively impact blood sugar levels by triggering the release of stress hormones like cortisol.

- **Stress-Reduction Techniques**:
  - Mindfulness meditation
  - Deep-breathing exercises
  - Engaging in hobbies or activities you enjoy

  - Ensuring adequate sleep

By addressing stress, you can improve not only your mental well-being but also your physical health.

Your Path Forward

Understanding the science behind the diabetic diet empowers you to make informed decisions about your health. Remember, managing diabetes is a journey, and you're not alone. Embrace the process of discovering new foods, recipes, and habits that contribute to a healthier, happier you.

Foods Diabetics Can Enjoy

Managing diabetes doesn't mean giving up delicious food. In fact, embracing a variety of nutritious foods can make meal times enjoyable while keeping your blood sugar levels in check.

1. Non-Starchy Vegetables

Non-starchy vegetables are the cornerstone of a diabetes-friendly diet. They're low in calories and carbohydrates but high in fiber, vitamins, and minerals. These veggies add volume to your meals without significantly impacting blood sugar, aiding in weight management and satiety.

Examples: Spinach, kale, broccoli, cauliflower, zucchini, bell peppers, cucumbers, asparagus.

In this cookbook, you'll find creative recipes that incorporate non-starchy vegetables into flavorful dishes—ranging from vibrant salads to hearty stir-fries—ensuring you get essential nutrients while maintaining stable glucose levels.

2. Lean Proteins

Protein plays a vital role in managing blood sugar by slowing the absorption of carbohydrates. Lean protein sources are low in unhealthy fats and provide essential amino acids for muscle maintenance and overall health.

Examples: Skinless chicken breast, turkey, lean cuts of beef, fish (salmon, cod, tuna), tofu, eggs.

My recipes often feature lean proteins paired with wholesome ingredients, creating balanced meals that are both nourishing and satisfying.

3. Whole Grains

Whole grains are rich in fiber and complex carbohydrates, which digest slowly and lead to a gradual rise in blood sugar levels. Unlike refined grains, whole grains retain their nutrient-rich bran and germ layers.

Examples: Quinoa, brown rice, whole oats, barley, bulgur, farro.

You'll discover a variety of recipes that incorporate whole grains—from hearty breakfasts to wholesome side dishes—providing energy and keeping you fuller longer without causing sharp glucose spikes.

4. Healthy Fats

Incorporating healthy fats into your diet can improve heart health and enhance the flavor of your meals. These fats help you feel satiated and can slow the digestion of carbohydrates, promoting more stable blood sugar levels.

Examples: Olive oil, avocados, nuts (almonds, walnuts), seeds (chia seeds, flaxseeds), fatty fish (salmon, mackerel).

The recipes in this book balance healthy fats with other nutrient-dense ingredients, ensuring each meal supports your health while delighting your palate.

5. Low-Glycemic Fruits

Fruits with a low glycemic index (GI) can be enjoyed in moderation, providing natural sweetness along with fiber, vitamins, and antioxidants. These fruits have a minimal impact on blood sugar compared to high-GI fruits.

Examples: Berries (strawberries, blueberries), apples, pears, grapefruit, cherries.

I've included delightful ways to incorporate these fruits into your diet—such as smoothies, salads, and desserts—allowing you to indulge your sweet tooth without compromising blood sugar control.

6. Legumes

Legumes are nutritional powerhouses packed with fiber, protein, and essential nutrients. They help stabilize blood sugar levels and keep you feeling full, making them an excellent addition to a diabetic diet.

Examples: Lentils, chickpeas, black beans, kidney beans.

In this cookbook, legumes feature prominently in soups, stews, and salads, offering versatile and satisfying options that support both glucose management and digestive health.

Additional Insights

Exploring Herbs and Spices

Enhance the flavor of your meals without adding extra sugar or salt by using herbs and spices. Ingredients like cinnamon, turmeric, garlic, and rosemary not only add depth to your dishes but also offer health benefits, such as anti-inflammatory properties.

The Importance of Hydration

Staying hydrated aids in regulating blood sugar levels and supports overall bodily functions. Aim to drink plenty of water throughout the day, and consider herbal teas or infused waters with slices of citrus or cucumber for added flavor.

Fermented Foods for Gut Health

Incorporating fermented foods like yogurt, kefir, sauerkraut, and kimchi can promote a healthy gut microbiome, which may positively influence blood sugar control and immune function.

Mindful Eating Practices

Paying attention to your hunger and fullness cues can prevent overeating. Eating slowly and savoring each bite not only enhances your enjoyment of food but also allows your body time to signal when it's satisfied, aiding in portion control.

Foods to Limit or Avoid for Diabetics

Managing diabetes effectively involves not just knowing what to eat but also understanding which foods can hinder your progress. In **"The Complete Diabetic Cookbook for Beginners,"** I, **Linette Johnston**, shed light on foods that those with diabetes should limit or avoid to maintain optimal health and stable blood sugar levels.

1. Sugary Foods and Beverages

High-sugar foods and drinks can cause rapid spikes in blood glucose, making them less than ideal for diabetes management. These aren't limited to obvious sweets but also include items with hidden sugars.

Examples: Soda, energy drinks, sweetened fruit juices, candies, cakes, cookies, sugary cereals.

In this cookbook, I focus on minimizing added sugars while offering delicious alternatives. You'll find naturally sweetened recipes and those using sugar substitutes like stevia, allowing you to enjoy treats without the glucose surge.

2. Refined Carbohydrates

Refined carbs lack fiber and essential nutrients due to processing, leading to quick digestion and sharp increases in blood sugar.

Examples: White bread, regular pasta, white rice, pastries, bagels, many crackers.

I encourage swapping out refined grains for whole grains or low-carb alternatives. My recipes help you maintain balanced blood sugar without sacrificing taste, using ingredients like quinoa, whole-grain bread, and zucchini noodles.

3. Trans Fats

Trans fats, often found in processed and fried foods, not only affect blood sugar but also increase the risk of heart disease—a significant concern for diabetics.

Examples: Fried fast foods, certain packaged snacks (some chips and crackers), margarine, processed baked goods like pies and donuts.

My recipes prioritize heart-healthy fats such as olive oil, avocados, and nuts. By avoiding trans fats, you support cardiovascular health while enjoying flavorful meals.

4. Processed Meats

Processed meats are typically high in unhealthy fats, sodium, and preservatives, which can contribute to hypertension and inflammation—factors that complicate diabetes management.

Examples: Sausages, bacon, hot dogs, deli meats, salami.

In "The Complete Diabetic Cookbook for Beginners," I focus on fresh, lean proteins like chicken, turkey, and plant-based options. This ensures your meals are nutritious and lower in harmful additives, yet rich in flavor.

5. Sweetened Dairy Products

While dairy can be part of a healthy diet, sweetened versions add unnecessary sugars that can spike blood glucose levels.

Examples: Flavored yogurts, sweetened milks (including some plant-based milks), ice cream, sweetened condensed milk.

I incorporate unsweetened dairy products and suggest natural flavor enhancers like fresh fruit or vanilla extract. This way, you can enjoy creamy textures without the added sugars.

6. Highly Processed Snack Foods

Processed snacks often contain a mix of unhealthy fats, sugars, and refined carbs, offering little nutritional value and causing quick blood sugar elevations.

Examples: Potato chips, pretzels, packaged cookies, sugary granola bars, microwave popcorn with added butter and salt.

My cookbook offers healthier snack alternatives, such as roasted chickpeas, spiced nuts, and vegetable sticks with hummus, keeping you satisfied between meals without compromising your health.

Additional Insights

Alcohol Consumption

Alcohol can interfere with blood sugar levels and insulin effectiveness. It can cause both high and low blood sugar episodes, depending on the amount consumed and whether it's accompanied by food.

Tip: If you choose to drink alcohol, do so in moderation and always with a meal. Opt for dry wines or spirits mixed with sugar-free mixers, and monitor your blood sugar levels closely.

Hidden Sugars in Condiments

Many condiments and sauces are surprisingly high in added sugars, which can add up quickly and impact your glucose control.

Examples: Ketchup, barbecue sauce, certain salad dressings, sweet chili sauce.

Tip: Read labels carefully and consider making your own condiments at home. In the cookbook, you'll find recipes for low-sugar dressings and sauces that are both tasty and diabetes-friendly.

Beware of "Fat-Free" Labels

Products labeled as "fat-free" or "low-fat" often compensate with added sugars to enhance flavor.

Examples: Fat-free yogurt, low-fat peanut butter, reduced-fat cookies.

Tip: Choose whole foods when possible and don't rely solely on labeling. Check the nutritional information to make informed choices.

Sodium Intake Matters

Excessive sodium can lead to high blood pressure, further increasing the risk of heart disease and stroke for those with diabetes.

Examples: Canned soups, instant noodles, processed meats, salted snacks.

Tip: Opt for low-sodium versions of products and season your food with herbs and spices instead of salt. Homemade soups and broths from my cookbook allow you to control the sodium content effectively.

By being mindful of these foods and making strategic substitutions, you can enjoy a diverse and satisfying diet while effectively managing your diabetes. **"The Complete Diabetic Cookbook for Beginners"** is designed to guide you through making healthier choices without feeling deprived, turning potential dietary restrictions into culinary opportunities

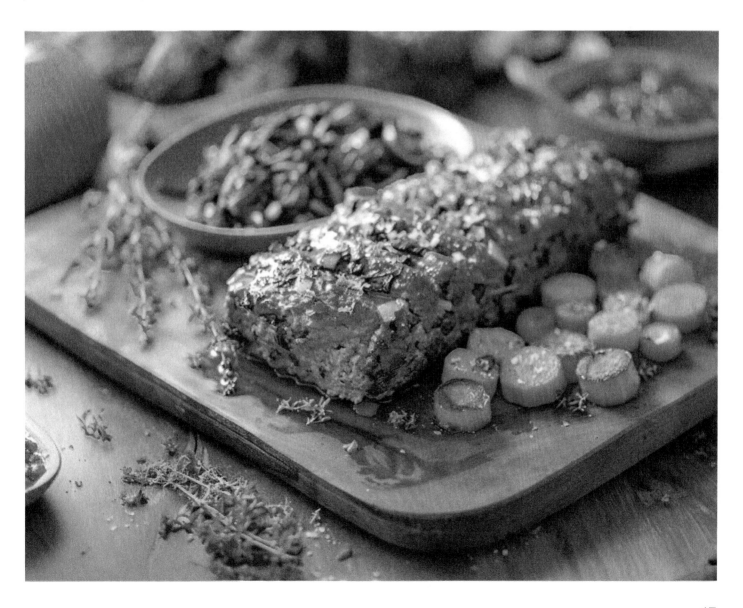

CHAPTER 2: 30-DAY MEAL PLAN

Day	Breakfast (400 kcal)	Lunch (500 kcal)	Snack (220 kcal)	Dinner (380 kcal)
Day 1	Spinach and Avocado Smoothie - p.26	Chickpea and Spinach Curry - p.37	Almond Flour Blueberry Muffins - p.57	Grilled Salmon with Asparagus - p.69
Day 2	Zucchini and Cheese Frittata - p.21	Ground Turkey and Vegetable Casserole - p.47	Cucumber Slices with Hummus - p.49	Baked Cod with Lemon and Dill - p.69
Day 3	Cottage Cheese with Sliced Almonds and Blueberries - p.23	Farro and Roasted Vegetable Bowl - p.38	Low-Carb Lemon Cheesecake Bars - p.53	Eggplant Lasagna with Ricotta - p.73
Day 4	Turkey and Cheese Roll-ups - p.30	Grilled Chicken and Veggie Bowl - p.41	Greek Yogurt with Cucumbers - p.50	Herb-Crusted Tilapia - p.70
Day 5	Chia Seed Pudding with Almond Milk and Nuts - p.22	Beef and Barley Stew - p.36	Zucchini and Feta Stuffed Mushrooms - p.51	Pesto-Crusted Salmon with Vegetables - p.72
Day 6	Veggie Egg Muffins - p.20	Quinoa and Black Bean Salad with Avocado - p.38	Low-Carb Chocolate Chip Cookies - p.55	Braised Cod with Tomatoes and Spinach - p.75
Day 7	Almond Butter and Banana Smoothie - p.26	Wild Rice with Cauliflower and Chicken Burrito - p.40	Eggplant Rolls with Nut Stuffing - p.50	Grilled Tuna Steaks with Avocado Salsa - p.71
Day 8	Zucchini and Mushroom Egg Bake - p.25	Chicken and Turkey Cutlets - p.44	Vanilla Chia Seed Pudding - p.52	Baked Halibut with Roasted Vegetables - p.71
Day 9	Breakfast Burrito with Lettuce Wrap - p.21	Stuffed Cabbage Rolls with Ground Turkey and Quinoa - p.39	Coconut Flour Brownies - p.52	Mahi Mahi Tacos with Cabbage Slaw - p.70
Day 10	Spinach and Feta Stuffed Peppers - p.24	Kale and Chicken Caesar Salad - p.42	Sliced Bell Peppers with Guacamole - p.49	Roasted Cauliflower Steaks with Chimichurri Sauce - p.65
Day 11	Buckwheat Porridge with Mushrooms and Cheese - p.29	Zucchini Noodles with Pesto Chicken - p.43	Low-Carb Tiramisu - p.53	Grilled Swordfish with Herb Butter and Cauliflower - p.74
Day 12	Mushroom and Swiss Cheese Omelette - p.23	Chicken and Avocado Salad - p.44	Lemon Coconut Balls - p.56	Asian-Inspired Chicken Salad with Sesame Dressing - p.67
Day 13	Quinoa Breakfast Bowl with Orange Zest and Almonds - p.28	Broccoli and Turkey Meatball Lunch Box - p.43	Low-Carb Pumpkin Pie - p.56	Tilapia with Mango Salsa - p.75
Day 14	Turkey Sausage and Pepper Breakfast Bake - p.31	Brown Rice Pilaf - p.37	Almond Flour Raspberry Bars - p.59	Buckwheat and Roasted Pumpkin Salad - p.68
Day 15	Spinach and Ricotta Crepes - p.33	Hearty Lentil and Spinach Soup - p.35	Artichoke and Spinach Yogurt Dip with Eggplant - p.51	Baked Sole with Lemon and Capers - p.72
Day 16	Keto Pancakes with Almond Flour and Cream Cheese Filling - p.33	Meatballs with Couscous - p.46	Low-Carb Banana Nut Muffins - p.58	Warm Lentil and Roasted Veggie Salad - p.64

Day	Breakfast (400 kcal)	Lunch (500 kcal)	Snack (220 kcal)	Dinner (380 kcal)
Day 17	Avocado and Spinach Omelette - p.20	Quinoa Paella - p.74	Chocolate Avocado Pudding - p.54	Grilled Green Beans with Lemon Zest and Mushrooms - p.63
Day 18	Zucchini Fritters with Sour Cream - p.32	Roasted Veggie and Hummus Wrap - p.41	Vanilla Almond Protein Bars - p.54	Herb-Crusted Tilapia - p.70
Day 19	Low-Carb Breakfast Casserole - p.22	Beef and Barley Stew - p.36	Almond Flour Snickerdoodle Cookies - p.60	Salmon, Shrimp, and Avocado Salad - p.73
Day 20	Carrot and Ginger Smoothie - p.27	Farro and Roasted Vegetable Bowl - p.38	Raspberry Almond Tarts - p.55	Baked Cod with Lemon and Dill - p.69
Day 21	Chicken and Spinach Breakfast Wrap - p.31	Chickpea and Spinach Stuffed Acorn Squash - p.64	Greek Yogurt with Cucumbers - p.50	Eggplant and Lentil Salad with Mint Yogurt Dressing - p.63
Day 22	Oatmeal with Sliced Bananas and Walnuts - p.24	Turkey Meatloaf with Spinach and Roasted Vegetables - p.45	Sugar-Free Lemon Poppy Seed Muffins - p.59	Grilled Salmon with Asparagus - p.69
Day 23	Almond Flour Waffles with Avocado and Smoked Salmon - p.32	Quinoa and Black Bean Salad with Avocado - p.38	Low-Carb Lemon Cheesecake Bars - p.53	Spinach and Grilled Chicken Salad with Avocado - p.66
Day 24	Cauliflower and Ham Breakfast Casserole - p.25	Grilled Chicken and Veggie Bowl - p.41	Zucchini and Feta Stuffed Mushrooms - p.51	Pesto-Crusted Salmon with Vegetables - p.72
Day 25	Orange and Spinach Smoothie - p.27	Stuffed Cabbage Rolls with Ground Turkey and Quinoa - p.39	Coconut Flour Brownies - p.52	Eggplant Lasagna with Ricotta - p.73
Day 26	Bacon and Avocado Salad - p.30	Zucchini Noodles with Pesto Chicken - p.43	Low-Carb Chocolate Chip Cookies - p.55	Roasted Beetroot and Quinoa Salad with Feta Cheese - p.68
Day 27	Keto Breakfast Pizza - p.34	Chicken and Avocado Salad - p.44	Lemon Pound Cake with Almond Flour - p.61	Herb-Crusted Tilapia - p.70
Day 28	Zucchini and Mushroom Egg Bake - p.25	Broccoli and Turkey Meatball Lunch Box - p.43	Sliced Bell Peppers with Guacamole - p.49	Grilled Tuna Steaks with Avocado Salsa - p.71
Day 29	Veggie Egg Muffins - p.20	Kale and Chicken Caesar Salad - p.42	Low-Carb Tiramisu - p.53	Baked Halibut with Roasted Vegetables - p.71
Day 30	Mushroom and Swiss Cheese Omelette - p.23	Ground Turkey and Vegetable Casserole - p.47	Eggplant Rolls with Nut Stuffing - p.50	Mahi Mahi Tacos with Cabbage Slaw - p.70

Note: The 30-Day Meal Plan provided is intended as a flexible guide and source of inspiration. Calorie counts are approximate and may vary based on portion sizes and specific ingredients. We've crafted this plan to offer a diverse, balanced menu rich in proteins, healthy fats, and carbohydrates, allowing you to enjoy nutritious meals without sacrificing flavor.

If the caloric content doesn't fully match your personal needs, feel free to adjust the portion sizes. Modify the recipes to suit your individual goals and preferences. Be creative and enjoy each dish in a way that works best for you!

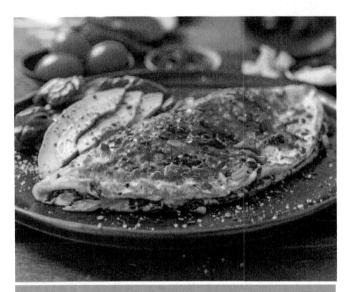

Avocado and Spinach Omelette

Prep: 10 mins | Cook: 10 mins | Serves: 2

Ingredients:

- 4 large eggs (200g)
- 1/2 cup diced avocado (75g)
- 1 cup fresh spinach, chopped (30g)
- 1/4 cup shredded cheddar cheese (30g)
- 1 tbsp olive oil (15ml)
- 1/4 tsp salt (1.5g)
- 1/4 tsp black pepper (1.5g)

Instructions:

1. Whisk eggs in a bowl with salt and pepper.
2. Heat olive oil in a non-stick skillet.
3. Add spinach to the skillet and cook until wilted.
4. Pour eggs over spinach and cook until edges start to set, about 3 minutes.
5. Sprinkle avocado and cheese on one half of the omelette.
6. Fold the omelette in half and cook until cheese melts, about 2-3 minutes.

Nutritional Facts (Per Serving): Calories: 400 | Sugars: 2g | Fat: 17g | Carbohydrates: 6g | Protein: 23g | Fiber: 4g | Sodium: 350mg

Glycemic Index: Eggs: Negligible GI (no carbs) | Avocado: Low (GI = 15) | Spinach: Low (GI = 15) | Cheddar Cheese: Negligible GI (no carbs)

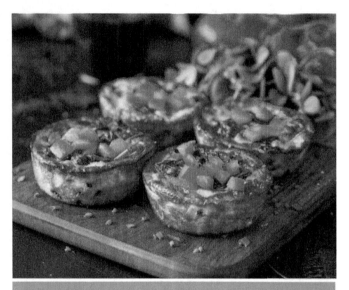

Veggie Egg Muffins

Prep: 15 mins | Cook: 20 mins | Serves: 6

Ingredients:

- 6 large eggs (300g)
- 1/2 cup diced bell peppers (75g)
- 1/2 cup diced tomatoes (75g)
- 1/2 cup chopped spinach (15g)
- 1/4 cup shredded cheddar cheese (30g)
- 1/4 cup Greek yogurt (60g)
- 1/2 tsp salt (3g)
- 1/4 tsp black pepper (1.5g)

Instructions:

1. Preheat oven to 375°F (190°C).
2. In a large bowl, whisk together eggs, Greek yogurt, salt, and pepper.
3. Stir in bell peppers, tomatoes, spinach, and cheese.
4. Grease a muffin tin and pour the mixture evenly into 6 cups.
5. Bake for 20 minutes or until the eggs are set.
6. Let cool slightly before serving.

Nutritional Facts (Per Serving): Calories: 400 | Sugars: 4g | Fat: 13g | Carbohydrates: 5g | Protein: 20g | Fiber: 2g | Sodium: 400mg

Glycemic Index: Eggs: Negligible GI (no carbs) | Bell Peppers: Low (GI = 15) | Tomatoes: Low (GI = 15) | Spinach: Low (GI = 15) | Cheddar Cheese: Negligible GI (no carbs) | Greek Yogurt: Low (GI = 15)

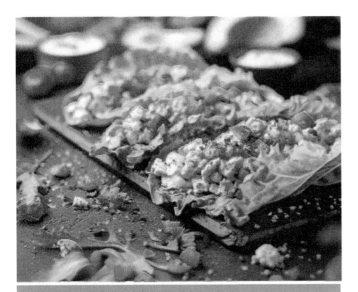

Breakfast Burrito with Lettuce Wrap

Prep: 10 mins | Cook: 10 mins | Serves: 2

Ingredients:

- 4 large eggs (200g)
- 1/2 cup diced bell peppers (75g)
- 1/2 cup diced tomatoes (75g)
- 1/4 cup shredded cheddar cheese (30g)
- 1/4 cup Greek yogurt (60g)
- 2 large lettuce leaves (50g)
- 1 tbsp olive oil (15ml)
- 1/4 tsp salt (1.5g)
- 1/4 tsp black pepper (1.5g)

Instructions:

1. Whisk eggs with salt and pepper.
2. Heat olive oil in a non-stick skillet over medium heat.
3. Add bell peppers and tomatoes, sauté for 2 minutes.
4. Pour eggs into the skillet and scramble until cooked through, about 5 minutes.
5. Stir in cheddar cheese until melted.
6. Spoon the egg mixture onto the lettuce leaves and top with Greek yogurt.
7. Roll the lettuce leaves to form wraps.

Nutritional Facts (Per Serving): Calories: 400 | Sugars: 4g | Fat: 15g | Carbohydrates: 6g | Protein: 23g | Fiber: 2g | Sodium: 350mg

Glycemic Index: Eggs: Negligible GI (no carbs) | Bell Peppers: Low (GI = 15) | Tomatoes: Low (GI = 15) | Lettuce: Low (GI = 10) | Cheddar Cheese: Negligible GI (no carbs) | Greek Yogurt: Low (GI = 15)

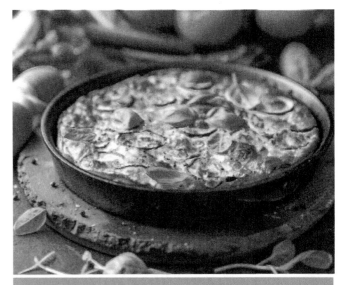

Zucchini and Cheese Frittata

Prep: 10 mins | Cook: 20 mins | Serves: 2

Ingredients:

- 4 large eggs (200g)
- 1 cup grated zucchini (150g)
- 1/4 cup shredded mozzarella cheese (30g)
- 1/4 cup Greek yogurt (60g)
- 1 tbsp olive oil (15ml)
- 1/4 tsp salt (1.5g)
- 1/4 tsp black pepper (1.5g)

Instructions:

1. Preheat oven to 375°F (190°C).
2. Whisk eggs with Greek yogurt, salt, and pepper.
3. Heat olive oil in an oven-safe skillet over medium heat.
4. Add grated zucchini and cook until softened, about 3 minutes.
5. Pour egg mixture over zucchini and cook until edges start to set, about 5 minutes.
6. Sprinkle mozzarella cheese on top.
7. Transfer skillet to oven and bake until the frittata is fully set, about 10-12 minutes.

Nutritional Facts (Per Serving): Calories: 400 | Sugars: 5g | Fat: 16g | Carbohydrates: 7g | Protein: 22g | Fiber: 2g | Sodium: 350mg

Glycemic Index: Eggs: Negligible GI (no carbs) | Zucchini: Low (GI = 15) | Mozzarella Cheese: Negligible GI (no carbs) | Greek Yogurt: Low (GI = 15)

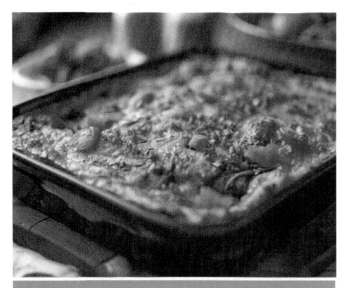

Low-carb Breakfast Casserole

Prep: 15 mins | Cook: 35 mins | Serves: 2

Ingredients:

- 4 large eggs (200g)
- 1 cup chopped spinach (30g)
- 1/2 cup diced bell peppers (75g)
- 1/2 cup diced tomatoes (75g)
- 1/4 cup shredded cheddar cheese (30g)
- 1/4 cup Greek yogurt (60g)
- 1 tbsp olive oil (15ml)
- 1/2 tsp salt (3g)
- 1/4 tsp black pepper (1.5g)

Instructions:

1. Preheat oven to 375°F (190°C).
2. Whisk eggs, Greek yogurt, salt, and pepper in a large bowl. Heat olive oil in a skillet.
3. Add bell peppers and tomatoes, cook for 3-4 minutes until softened. Stir in spinach and cook until wilted, about 2 minutes. Transfer vegetables to a greased baking dish.
4. Pour the egg mixture over the vegetables and sprinkle with cheddar cheese.
5. Bake for 25-30 minutes, or until the eggs are set.

Nutritional Facts (Per Serving): Calories: 400 | Sugars: 5g | Fat: 15g | Carbohydrates: 10g | Protein: 22g | Fiber: 3g | Sodium: 450mg

Glycemic Index: Eggs: Negligible GI (no carbs) | Spinach: Low (GI = 15) | Bell Peppers: Low (GI = 15) | Tomatoes: Low (GI = 15) | Cheddar Cheese: Negligible GI (no carbs) | Greek Yogurt: Low (GI = 15)

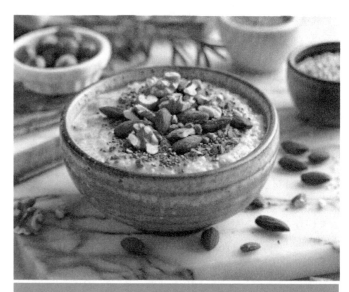

Chia Seed Pudding with Unsweetened Almond Milk

Prep: 5 mins | Cook: Chill for 4 hours | Serves: 2

Ingredients:

- 1/4 cup chia seeds (40g)
- 1 cup unsweetened almond milk (240ml)
- 1 tbsp low carb sweetener (12g)
- 1/2 tsp vanilla extract (2.5ml)
- 1/4 cup chopped nuts (30g)

Instructions:

1. In a bowl, combine chia seeds, almond milk, low carb sweetener, and vanilla extract.
2. Stir well to mix and let sit for 5 minutes. Stir again to prevent clumping.
3. Cover and refrigerate for at least 4 hours or overnight.
4. Stir before serving and top with chopped nuts.

Nutritional Facts (Per Serving): Calories: 400 | Sugars: 2g | Fat: 17g | Carbohydrates: 40g | Protein: 10g | Fiber: 8g | Sodium: 150mg

Glycemic Index: Chia Seeds: Low (GI = 1) | Almond Milk: Low (GI = 30) | Nuts: Low (GI = 15) | Low Carb Sweetener: Negligible GI | Vanilla Extract: Negligible GI

CHAPTER 4: BREAKFASTS: Quick And Easy Breakfast Ideas

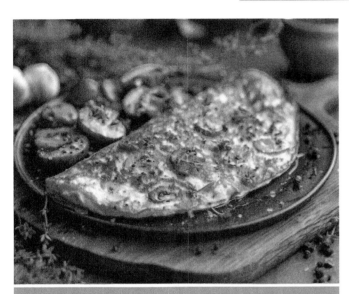

Mushroom and Swiss Cheese Omelette

Prep: 10 mins | Cook: 10 mins | Serves: 2

Ingredients:

- 4 large eggs (200g)
- 1/2 cup sliced mushrooms (50g)
- 1/4 cup shredded Swiss cheese (30g)
- 1/4 cup Greek yogurt (60g)
- 1 tbsp olive oil (15ml)
- 1/4 tsp salt (1.5g)
- 1/4 tsp black pepper

Instructions:

1. Whisk eggs with Greek yogurt, salt, and pepper.
2. Heat olive oil in a non-stick skillet.
3. Add mushrooms and sauté about 3-4 minutes.
4. Pour egg mixture into the skillet and cook until edges start to set, about 3 minutes.
5. Sprinkle Swiss cheese over half of the omelette.
6. Fold the omelette in half and cook until cheese melts, about 2-3 minutes.

Nutritional Facts (Per Serving): Calories: 400 | Sugars: 2g | Fat: 17g | Carbohydrates: 5g | Protein: 23g | Fiber: 1g | Sodium: 400mg

Glycemic Index: Eggs: Negligible GI (no carbs) | Mushrooms: Low (GI = 15) | Swiss Cheese: Negligible GI (no carbs) | Greek Yogurt: Low (GI = 15)

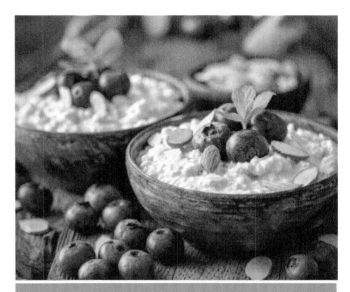

Cottage Cheese with Sliced Almonds and Blueberries

Prep: 5 mins | Cook: None | Serves: 2

Ingredients:

- 1 cup cottage cheese (240g)
- 1/4 cup sliced almonds (30g)
- 1/2 cup fresh blueberries (75g)
- 1 tbsp low carb sweetener (12g)

Instructions:

1. Divide cottage cheese into two bowls.
2. Top each bowl with sliced almonds and fresh blueberries.
3. Sprinkle with low carb sweetener.

Nutritional Facts (Per Serving): Calories: 400 | Sugars: 5g | Fat: 15g | Carbohydrates: 20g | Protein: 23g | Fiber: 4g | Sodium: 450mg

Glycemic Index: Cottage Cheese: Low (GI = 30) | Almonds: Low (GI = 15) | Blueberries: Low (GI = 53) | Low Carb Sweetener: Negligible GI

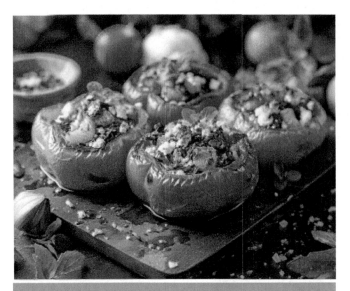

Spinach and Feta Stuffed Peppers

Prep: 15 mins | Cook: 25 mins | Serves: 2

Ingredients:

- 2 large bell peppers, halved and seeded (300g)
- 1 cup chopped spinach (30g)
- 1/2 cup crumbled feta cheese (75g)
- 1/4 cup Greek yogurt (60g)
- 1/4 cup diced onions (40g)
- 1 tbsp olive oil (15ml)
- 1/2 tsp salt (3g)
- 1/4 tsp black pepper (1.5g)

Instructions:

1. Preheat oven to 375°F (190°C).
2. Heat olive oil in a skillet over medium heat.
3. Add diced onions and cook until softened, about 3-4 minutes.
4. Stir in spinach and cook until wilted, about 2 minutes.
5. Remove from heat and mix in feta cheese, Greek yogurt, salt, and pepper.
6. Stuff each bell pepper half with the spinach mixture.
7. Place stuffed peppers in a baking dish and bake for 20-25 minutes until peppers are tender.

Nutritional Facts (Per Serving): Calories: 400 | Sugars: 5g | Fat: 16g | Carbohydrates: 17g | Protein: 15g | Fiber: 4g | Sodium: 550mg

Glycemic Index: Bell Peppers: Low (GI = 15) | Spinach: Low (GI = 15) | Feta Cheese: Low (GI = 34) | Greek Yogurt: Low (GI = 15) | Onions: Low (GI = 15)

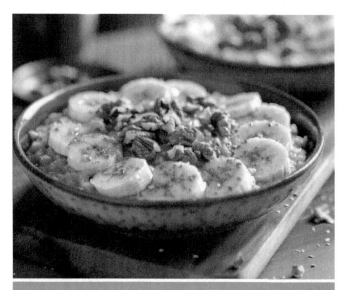

Oatmeal with Sliced Bananas and Walnuts

Prep: 5 mins | Cook: 10 mins | Serves: 2

Ingredients:

- 1 cup rolled oats (90g)
- 2 cups water or unsweetened almond milk (480ml)
- 1 medium banana, sliced (120g)
- 1/4 cup chopped walnuts (30g)
- 1 tbsp low carb sweetener (12g)
- 1/2 tsp cinnamon (2g)

Instructions:

1. In a pot, bring water or almond milk to a boil.
2. Add rolled oats and reduce heat to a simmer. Cook for 5-7 minutes, stirring occasionally.
3. Stir in low carb sweetener and cinnamon.
4. Divide oatmeal into two bowls.
5. Top each bowl with sliced bananas and chopped walnuts.

Nutritional Facts (Per Serving): Calories: 400 | Sugars: 6g | Fat: 17g | Carbohydrates: 40g | Protein: 10g | Fiber: 7g | Sodium: 10mg

Glycemic Index: Rolled Oats: Moderate (GI = 55) | Banana: Moderate (GI = 51) | Walnuts: Low (GI = 15) | Low Carb Sweetener: Negligible GI | Cinnamon: Negligible GI

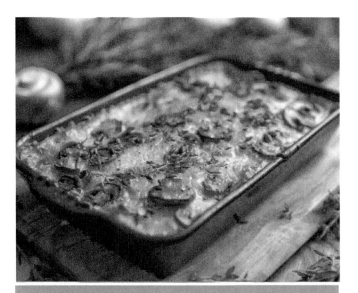

Zucchini and Mushroom Egg Bake

Prep: 15 mins | Cook: 30 mins | Serves: 2

Ingredients:

- 4 large eggs (200g)
- 1 cup grated zucchini (150g)
- 1/2 cup sliced mushrooms (50g)
- 1/4 cup shredded cheddar cheese (30g)
- 1/4 cup Greek yogurt (60g)
- 1 tbsp olive oil (15ml)
- 1/2 tsp salt (3g)
- 1/4 tsp black pepper (1.5g)

Instructions:

1. Preheat oven to 375°F (190°C).
2. In a bowl, whisk eggs, Greek yogurt, salt, and pepper.
3. Heat olive oil in a skillet over medium heat.
4. Add zucchini and mushrooms, cook for 3-4 minutes until softened.
5. Transfer vegetables to a greased baking dish.
6. Pour the egg mixture over the vegetables and sprinkle with cheddar cheese.
7. Bake for 20-25 minutes, or until eggs are set.

Nutritional Facts (Per Serving): Calories: 400 | Sugars: 3g | Fat: 16g | Carbohydrates: 8g | Protein: 22g | Fiber: 2g | Sodium: 450mg

Glycemic Index: Zucchini: Low (GI = 15) | Mushrooms: Low (GI = 15) | Cheddar Cheese: Negligible GI (no carbs) | Greek Yogurt: Low (GI = 15)

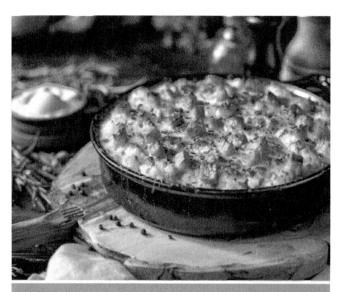

Cauliflower and Ham Breakfast Casserole

Prep: 15 mins | Cook: 35 mins | Serves: 2

Ingredients:

- 4 large eggs (200g)
- 1 cup riced cauliflower (100g)
- 1/2 cup diced ham (75g)
- 1/4 cup shredded Swiss cheese (30g)
- 1/4 cup Greek yogurt (60g)
- 1 tbsp olive oil (15ml)
- 1/2 tsp salt (3g)
- 1/4 tsp black pepper (1.5g)

Instructions:

1. Preheat oven to 375°F (190°C).
2. In a bowl, whisk eggs, Greek yogurt, salt, and pepper.
3. Heat olive oil in a skillet over medium heat.
4. Add riced cauliflower and cook for 5 minutes until slightly tender.
5. Stir in diced ham.
6. Transfer mixture to a greased baking dish.
7. Pour the egg mixture over the cauliflower and ham, and sprinkle with Swiss cheese.
8. Bake for 25-30 minutes, or until eggs are set.

Nutritional Facts (Per Serving): Calories: 400 | Sugars: 3g | Fat: 17g | Carbohydrates: 6g | Protein: 23g | Fiber: 2g | Sodium: 550mg

Glycemic Index: Cauliflower: Low (GI = 15) | Ham: Low (GI = 30) | Swiss Cheese: Negligible GI (no carbs) | Greek Yogurt: Low (GI = 15)

CHAPTER 5: BREAKFASTS: Nutrient-dense Smoothie Recipes

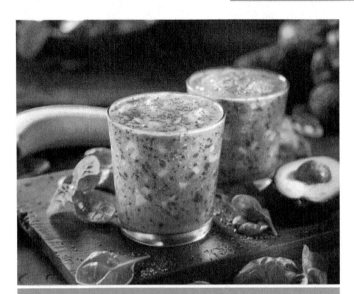

Spinach and Avocado Smoothie

Prep: 5 mins | Cook: None | Serves: 2

Ingredients:

- 1 cup unsweetened almond milk (240ml)
- 1 cup fresh spinach (30g)
- 1/2 ripe avocado (75g)
- 1/2 medium banana (60g)
- 1 tbsp low carb sweetener (12g)
- 1/2 tsp vanilla extract (2.5ml)
- 1/2 cup ice cubes (120g)

Instructions:

1. Combine all ingredients in a blender.
2. Blend until smooth.
3. Pour into glasses and serve.

Nutritional Facts (Per Serving): Calories: 400 | Sugars: 5g | Fat: 17g | Carbohydrates: 22g | Protein: 5g | Fiber: 8g | Sodium: 150mg

Glycemic Index: Spinach: Low (GI = 15) | Avocado: Low (GI = 15) | Banana: Moderate (GI = 51) | Almond Milk: Low (GI = 30)

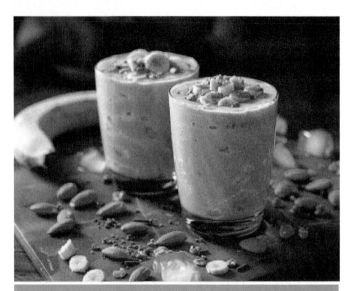

Almond Butter and Banana Smoothie

Prep: 5 mins | Cook: None | Serves: 2

Ingredients:

- 1 cup unsweetened almond milk (240ml)
- 2 tbsp almond butter (32g)
- 1 medium banana (120g)
- 1 tbsp low carb sweetener (12g)
- 1/2 tsp cinnamon (2g)
- 1/2 cup ice cubes (120g)

Instructions:

1. Combine all ingredients in a blender.
2. Blend until smooth.
3. Pour into glasses and serve.

Nutritional Facts (Per Serving): Calories: 400 | Sugars: 6g | Fat: 16g | Carbohydrates: 41g | Protein: 10g | Fiber: 6g | Sodium: 150mg

Glycemic Index: Almond Butter: Low (GI = 15) | Banana: Moderate (GI = 51) | Almond Milk: Low (GI = 30)

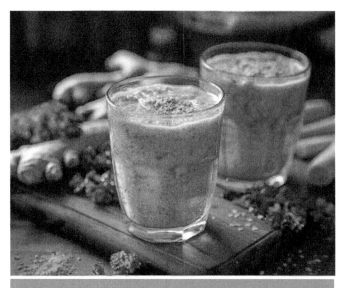

Carrot and Ginger Smoothie

Prep: 5 mins | Cook: None | Serves: 2

Ingredients:

- 1 cup unsweetened almond milk (240ml)
- 1 cup chopped carrots (130g)
- 1/2 inch fresh ginger, peeled and chopped (5g)
- 1 medium banana (120g)
- 1 tbsp low carb sweetener (12g)
- 1/2 cup ice cubes (120g)

Instructions:

1. Combine all ingredients in a blender.
2. Blend until smooth.
3. Pour into glasses and serve.

Nutritional Facts (Per Serving): Calories: 400 | Sugars: 6g | Fat: 14g | Carbohydrates: 47g | Protein: 6g | Fiber: 8g | Sodium: 105mg

Glycemic Index: Carrots: Moderate (GI = 41) | Ginger: Low (GI = 15) | Banana: Moderate (GI = 51) | Almond Milk: Low (GI = 30) | Low Carb Sweetener: Negligible GI

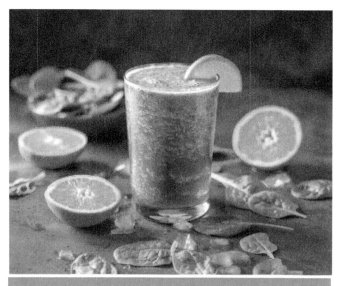

Orange and Spinach Smoothie

Prep: 5 mins | Cook: None | Serves: 2

Ingredients:

- 1 cup unsweetened almond milk (240ml)
- 1 medium orange, peeled and segmented (130g)
- 1 cup fresh spinach (30g)
- 1 medium banana (120g)
- 1 tbsp low carb sweetener (12g)
- 1/2 cup ice cubes (120g)

Instructions:

1. Combine all ingredients in a blender.
2. Blend until smooth.
3. Pour into glasses and serve.

Nutritional Facts (Per Serving): Calories: 400 | Sugars: 6g | Fat: 13g | Carbohydrates: 53g | Protein: 6g | Fiber: 8g | Sodium: 105mg

Glycemic Index: Orange: Moderate (GI = 43) | Spinach: Low (GI = 15) | Banana: Moderate (GI = 51) | Almond Milk: Low (GI = 30) | Low Carb Sweetener: Negligible GI

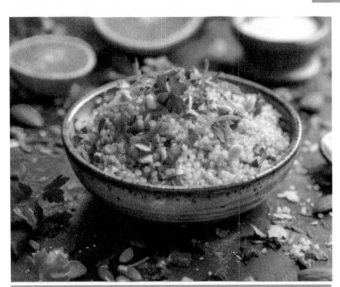

Quinoa Breakfast Bowl with Orange Zest and Almonds

Prep: 10 mins | Cook: 15 mins | Serves: 2

Ingredients:

- 1/2 cup quinoa (90g)
- 1 cup water (240ml)
- 1/2 cup chopped almonds (60g)
- 1 medium orange, zested (130g)
- 1 tbsp low carb sweetener (12g)
- 1/4 cup Greek yogurt (60g)
- 1/2 tsp cinnamon (2g)

Instructions:

1. In a pot, bring water to a boil, add quinoa, reduce heat, cover, and simmer for 15 minutes until tender.
2. Stir in chopped almonds, orange zest, low carb sweetener, Greek yogurt, and cinnamon.
3. Mix well and serve.

Nutritional Facts (Per Serving): Calories: 400 | Sugars: 5g | Fat: 17g | Carbohydrates: 40g | Protein: 14g | Fiber: 7g | Sodium: 50mg

Glycemic Index: Quinoa: Low (GI = 53) | Almonds: Low (GI = 15) | Orange: Moderate (GI = 43) | Greek Yogurt: Low (GI = 15) | Cinnamon: Negligible GI | Low Carb Sweetener: Negligible GI

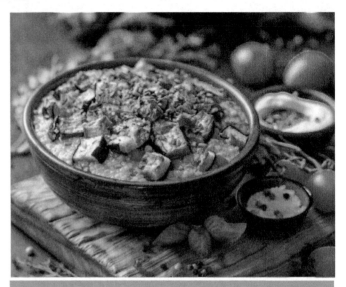

Amaranth Pudding with Cheese and Eggplant

Prep: 15 mins | Cook: 30 mins | Serves: 2

Ingredients:

- 1/2 cup amaranth (90g)
- 1 1/2 cups water (360ml)
- 1 cup diced eggplant (100g)
- 1/2 cup shredded mozzarella cheese (60g)
- 1/4 cup Greek yogurt (60g)
- 1 tbsp olive oil (15ml)
- 1/2 tsp salt (3g)
- 1/4 tsp black pepper (1.5g)

Instructions:

1. In a pot, bring water to a boil, add amaranth, reduce heat, cover, and simmer for 20 minutes until tender.
2. In a skillet, heat olive oil over medium heat. Add eggplant and cook until softened, about 5 minutes.
3. Stir eggplant into the cooked amaranth.
4. Mix in mozzarella cheese and Greek yogurt until well combined. Season with salt and pepper.

Nutritional Facts (Per Serving): Calories: 400 | Sugars: 3g | Fat: 15g | Carbohydrates: 48g | Protein: 20g | Fiber: 7g | Sodium: 450mg

Glycemic Index: Amaranth: Low (GI = 34) | Eggplant: Low (GI = 15) | Mozzarella Cheese: Low (GI = 34) | Greek Yogurt: Low (GI = 15)

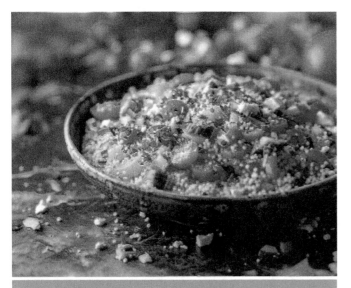

Couscous and Veggie Breakfast Bowl

Prep: 10 mins | Cook: 15 mins | Serves: 2

Ingredients:

- 1/2 cup couscous (90g)
- 1 cup water (240ml)
- 1/2 cup diced bell peppers (75g)
- 1/2 cup cherry tomatoes, halved (75g)
- 1/2 cup chopped cucumber (75g)
- 1/4 cup crumbled feta cheese (30g)
- 2 tbsp olive oil (30ml)
- 1 tbsp lemon juice (15ml)
- 1/4 tsp salt (1.5g)
- 1/4 tsp black pepper (1.5g)

Instructions:

1. Bring water to a boil, add couscous, cover, and remove from heat. Let it sit for 5 minutes. Fluff with a fork.
2. In a large bowl, combine couscous, bell peppers, cherry tomatoes, cucumber, and feta cheese.
3. In a small bowl, whisk together olive oil, lemon juice, salt, and pepper.
4. Pour the dressing over the couscous mixture and toss to combine.

Nutritional Facts (Per Serving): Calories: 400 | Sugars: 6g | Fat: 14g | Carbohydrates: 47g | Protein: 10g | Fiber: 6g | Sodium: 550mg

Glycemic Index: Couscous: Moderate (GI = 65) | Bell Peppers: Low (GI = 15) | Tomatoes: Low (GI = 15) | Cucumber: Low (GI = 15) | Feta Cheese: Low (GI = 34)

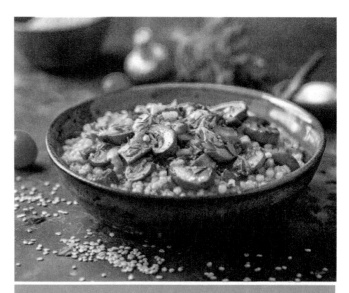

Buckwheat Porridge with Mushrooms and Cheese

Prep: 10 mins | Cook: 20 mins | Serves: 2

Ingredients:

- 1/2 cup buckwheat groats (90g)
- 1 1/2 cups water (360ml)
- 1 cup sliced mushrooms (100g)
- 1/2 cup shredded cheddar cheese (60g)
- 1/4 cup Greek yogurt (60g)
- 1 tbsp olive oil (15ml)
- 1/4 tsp salt (1.5g)
- 1/4 tsp black pepper (1.5g)

Instructions:

1. In a pot, bring water to a boil, add buckwheat groats, reduce heat, cover, and simmer for 15 minutes until tender.
2. In a skillet, heat olive oil over medium heat. Add mushrooms and cook until softened, about 5 minutes.
3. Stir mushrooms into the cooked buckwheat.
4. Mix in cheddar cheese and Greek yogurt until well combined. Season with salt and pepper.
5. Let the porridge sit for a few minutes to allow the flavors to meld.
6. Garnish with fresh herbs like parsley or chives before serving.

Nutritional Facts (Per Serving): Calories: 400 | Sugars: 3g | Fat: 14g | Carbohydrates: 47g | Protein: 20g | Fiber: 8g | Sodium: 450mg

Glycemic Index: Buckwheat: Low (GI = 54) | Mushrooms: Low (GI = 15) | Cheddar Cheese: Low (GI = 34) | Greek Yogurt: Low (GI = 15)

CHAPTER 7: BREAKFASTS: Protein-packed Options

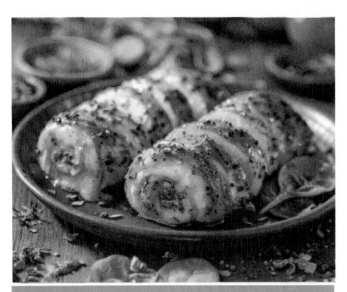

Turkey and Cheese Roll-ups

Prep: 10 mins | Cook: None | Serves: 2

Ingredients:

- 4 slices turkey breast (120g)
- 4 slices Swiss cheese (120g)
- 1/2 cup baby spinach (15g)
- 1/4 cup Greek yogurt (60g)
- 1 tbsp Dijon mustard (15g)
- 1/4 tsp black pepper (1.5g)

Instructions:

1. Lay out turkey slices on a flat surface.
2. Spread Greek yogurt evenly over turkey slices.
3. Add a slice of Swiss cheese on each turkey slice.
4. Place a handful of baby spinach on each slice.
5. Roll up each turkey slice tightly.
6. Secure with a toothpick if needed and serve.

Nutritional Facts (Per Serving): Calories: 400 | Sugars: 3g | Fat: 17g | Carbohydrates: 6g | Protein: 34g | Fiber: 1g | Sodium: 600mg

Glycemic Index: Turkey: Low (GI = 30) | Swiss Cheese: Low (GI = 34) | Spinach: Low (GI = 15) | Greek Yogurt: Low (GI = 15)

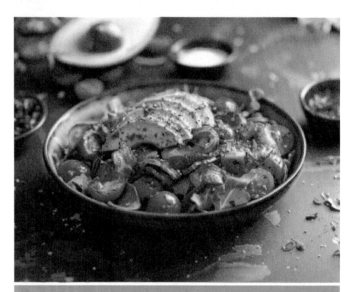

Bacon and Avocado Salad

Prep: 15 mins | Cook: None | Serves: 2

Ingredients:

- 4 slices bacon, cooked and crumbled (60g)
- 1 ripe avocado, diced (150g)
- 2 cups mixed greens (60g)
- 1/4 cup cherry tomatoes, halved (45g)
- 1/4 cup red onion, thinly sliced (30g)
- 2 tbsp olive oil (30ml)
- 1 tbsp lemon juice (15ml)
- 1/4 tsp salt (1.5g)
- 1/4 tsp black pepper (1.5g)

Instructions:

1. In a large bowl, combine mixed greens, cherry tomatoes, and red onion.
2. Add diced avocado and crumbled bacon.
3. In a small bowl, whisk together olive oil, lemon juice, salt, and pepper.
4. Drizzle the dressing over the salad and toss gently to combine.

Nutritional Facts (Per Serving): Calories: 400 | Sugars: 2g | Fat: 34g | Carbohydrates: 14g | Protein: 10g | Fiber: 8g | Sodium: 400mg

Glycemic Index: Bacon: Low (GI = 0) | Avocado: Low (GI = 15) | Mixed Greens: Low (GI = 15) | Cherry Tomatoes: Low (GI = 15) | Red Onion: Low (GI = 15)

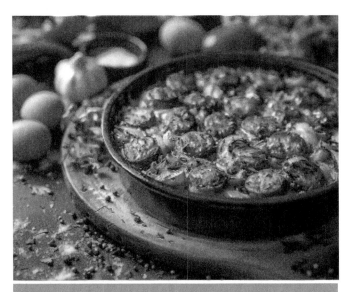

Turkey Sausage and Pepper Breakfast Bake

Prep: 15 mins | Cook: 30 mins | Serves: 2

Ingredients:

- 4 turkey sausages, sliced (200g)
- 1 cup diced bell peppers (150g)
- 1/2 cup diced onions (75g)
- 4 large eggs (200g)
- 1/4 cup shredded cheddar cheese (30g)
- 1/4 cup Greek yogurt (60g)
- 1 tbsp olive oil (15ml)
- 1/2 tsp salt (3g)
- 1/4 tsp black pepper (1.5g)

Instructions:

1. Preheat oven to 375°F (190°C).
2. In a skillet, heat olive oil over medium heat. Add turkey sausage slices and cook until browned, about 5 minutes.
3. Add diced bell peppers and onions, cook until softened, about 3-4 minutes. In a bowl, whisk eggs, Greek yogurt, salt, and pepper.
4. In a greased baking dish, combine sausage, peppers, onions, and egg mixture.
5. Sprinkle with shredded cheddar cheese.
6. Bake for 20-25 minutes, or until eggs are set.
7. Let cool slightly before serving.

Nutritional Facts (Per Serving): Calories: 400 | Sugars: 4g | Fat: 17g | Carbohydrates: 10g | Protein: 30g | Fiber: 2g | Sodium: 550mg

Glycemic Index: Turkey Sausage: Low (GI = 30) | Bell Peppers: Low (GI = 15) | Onions: Low (GI = 15) | Eggs: Negligible GI (no carbs) | Cheddar Cheese: Low (GI = 34) | Greek Yogurt: Low (GI = 15)

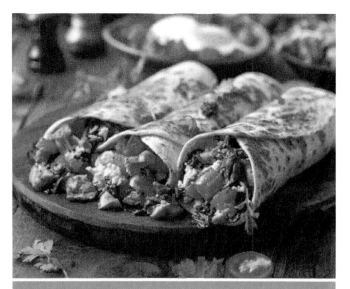

Chicken and Spinach Breakfast Wrap

Prep: 10 mins | Cook: 10 mins | Serves: 2

Ingredients:

- 4 large eggs (200g)
- 1 cup cooked, shredded chicken breast (150g)
- 1/2 cup diced tomatoes (75g)
- 1/4 cup shredded mozzarella cheese (30g)
- 1/4 cup Greek yogurt (60g)
- 2 whole wheat tortillas (120g)
- 1 tbsp olive oil (15ml)
- 1/2 tsp salt (3g)
- 1/4 tsp black pepper (1.5g)
- 1 cup fresh spinach (30g)

Instructions:

1. In a bowl, whisk eggs, salt, and pepper.
2. Heat olive oil in a skillet over medium heat. Add eggs and scramble until fully cooked, about 3-4 minutes.
3. Add shredded chicken, spinach, and diced tomatoes. Cook until spinach is wilted, about 2 minutes.
4. Remove from heat and stir in Greek yogurt and mozzarella cheese.
5. Divide the mixture evenly between the tortillas.
6. Roll up the tortillas and serve.

Nutritional Facts (Per Serving): Calories: 400 | Sugars: 4g | Fat: 14g | Carbohydrates: 40g | Protein: 30g | Fiber: 7g | Sodium: 600mg

Glycemic Index: Chicken: Low (GI = 30) | Spinach: Low (GI = 15) | Tomatoes: Low (GI = 15) | Mozzarella Cheese: Low (GI = 34) | Greek Yogurt: Low (GI = 15) | Whole Wheat Tortilla: Moderate (GI = 50)

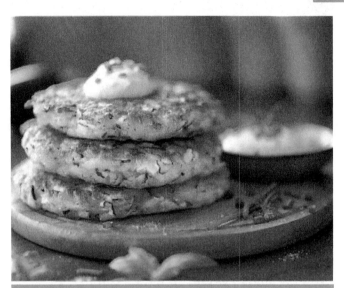

Zucchini Fritters with Sour Cream

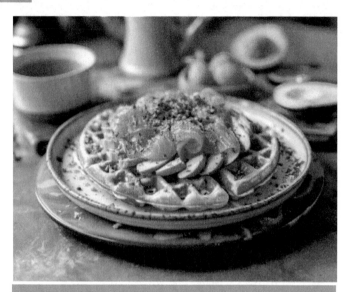

Almond Flour Waffles with Avocado and Smoked Salmon

Prep: 10 mins | Cook: 10 mins | Serves: 2

Ingredients:

- 2 cups grated zucchini (300g)
- 1/2 cup almond flour (50g)
- 1/4 cup chopped green onions (30g)
- 1/4 tsp salt (1.5g)
- 1/4 tsp black pepper (1.5g)
- 2 tbsp olive oil (30ml)
- 1/2 cup sour cream (120g)
- 2 large eggs (100g)

Instructions:

1. Grate zucchini and squeeze out excess moisture. In a bowl, mix zucchini, almond flour, eggs, green onions, salt, and pepper.
2. Heat olive oil in a skillet over medium heat.
3. Scoop 1/4 cup of the mixture for each fritter and flatten in the skillet. Cook for 3-4 minutes per side until golden brown.
4. Serve fritters with a dollop of sour cream.

Nutritional Facts (Per Serving): Calories: 400 | Sugars: 4g | Fat: 26g | Carbohydrates: 20g | Protein: 14g | Fiber: 6g | Sodium: 450mg

Glycemic Index: Zucchini: Low (GI = 15) | Almond Flour: Low (GI = 15) | Eggs: Negligible GI (no carbs) | Green Onions: Low (GI = 10) | Sour Cream: Low (GI = 30)

Prep: 10 mins | Cook: 15 mins | Serves: 2

Ingredients:

- 1 cup almond flour (100g)
- 4 large eggs (200g)
- 2 tbsp butter, for cooking (30g)
- 1 tbsp low carb sweetener (12g)
- 1/2 tsp baking powder (2g)
- 1/4 tsp salt (1.5g)
- 1 avocado, sliced (150g)
- 1/4 cup Greek yogurt (60g)
- 4 oz smoked salmon (120g)
- 1 tbsp lemon juice (15ml)

Instructions:

1. In a bowl, whisk together almond flour, eggs, Greek yogurt, low carb sweetener, baking powder, and salt.Preheat waffle iron and grease with butter.
2. Pour batter into the waffle iron and cook according to manufacturer's instructions until golden brown.
3. Top each waffle with sliced avocado and smoked salmon. Drizzle with lemon juice.

Nutritional Facts (Per Serving): Calories: 400 | Sugars: 2g | Fat: 30g | Carbohydrates: 10g | Protein: 20g | Fiber: 6g | Sodium: 450mg

Glycemic Index: Almond Flour: Low (GI = 15) | Eggs: Negligible GI (no carbs) | Greek Yogurt: Low (GI = 15) | Low Carb Sweetener: Negligible GI | Avocado: Low (GI = 15) | Smoked Salmon: Negligible GI (no carbs)

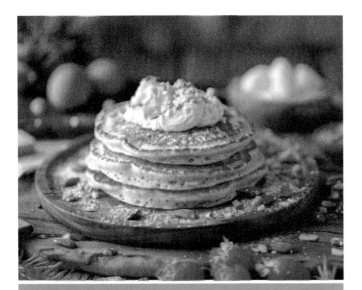

Keto Pancakes with Almond Flour and Cream Cheese Filling

Prep: 10 mins | Cook: 15 mins | Serves: 2

Ingredients:

- 1 cup almond flour (100g)
- 4 large eggs (200g)
- 1/4 cup Greek yogurt (60g)
- 1 tbsp low carb sweetener (12g)
- 1/2 tsp baking powder (2g)
- 1/4 tsp salt (1.5g)
- 1/4 cup cream cheese, softened (60g)
- 1 tsp vanilla extract (5ml)
- 2 tbsp butter, for cooking (30g)

Instructions:

1. Whisk together almond flour, eggs, Greek yogurt, sweetener, baking powder, salt, and vanilla extract.
2. Melt butter in a skillet over medium heat. Pour 1/4 cup of batter per pancake. Cook until bubbles form, flip, and cook the other side.
3. Soften cream cheese until smooth.
4. Spread cream cheese on each pancake and stack them.
5. Let them sit briefly to melt the filling. Optionally top with Greek yogurt, almond flour, or fresh berries.

Nutritional Facts (Per Serving): Calories: 400 | Sugars: 3g | Fat: 30g | Carbohydrates: 12g | Protein: 18g | Fiber: 5g | Sodium: 350mg

Glycemic Index: Almond Flour: Low (GI = 15) | Eggs: Negligible GI (no carbs) | Greek Yogurt: Low (GI = 15) | Low Carb Sweetener: Negligible GI | Cream Cheese: Low (GI = 34)

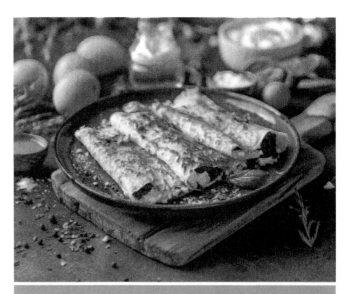

Spinach and Ricotta Crepes

Prep: 15 mins | Cook: 15 mins | Serves: 2

Ingredients:

- 1 cup almond flour (100g)
- 4 large eggs (200g)
- 1/4 cup Greek yogurt (60g)
- 1 tbsp low carb sweetener (12g)
- 1/2 cup ricotta cheese (125g)
- 1 cup fresh spinach, chopped (30g)
- 1/4 tsp salt (1.5g)
- 1/4 tsp black pepper (1.5g)
- 1 tbsp olive oil (15ml)

Instructions:

1. In a bowl, whisk together almond flour, eggs, Greek yogurt, low carb sweetener, and salt.
2. Heat a non-stick skillet over medium heat and add a small amount of olive oil.
3. Pour a small amount of batter into the skillet, swirling to coat the bottom thinly. Cook for 2-3 minutes per side until golden. Repeat with remaining batter.
4. In a separate bowl, mix ricotta cheese, chopped spinach, salt, and pepper.
5. Fill each crepe with the spinach and ricotta mixture and roll up.

Nutritional Facts (Per Serving): Calories: 400 | Sugars: 3g | Fat: 25g | Carbohydrates: 15g | Protein: 20g | Fiber: 6g | Sodium: 450mg

Glycemic Index: Almond Flour: Low (GI = 15) | Eggs: Negligible GI (no carbs) | Greek Yogurt: Low (GI = 15) | Ricotta Cheese: Low (GI = 27) | Spinach: Low (GI = 15)

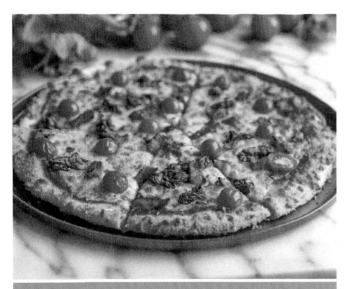

Keto Breakfast Pizza

Prep: 15 mins | Cook: 20 mins | Serves: 2

Ingredients:

- 1 cup almond flour (100g)
- 1/4 cup Greek yogurt (60g)
- 1/2 cup shredded mozzarella cheese (60g)
- 2 large eggs (100g)
- 1/2 cup cooked bacon, crumbled (60g)
- 1/2 cup cherry tomatoes, halved (75g)
- 1/4 cup chopped spinach (30g)
- 1 tbsp olive oil (15ml)
- 1/2 tsp baking powder (2g)
- 1/4 tsp salt (1.5g)
- 1/4 tsp black pepper (1.5g)

Instructions:

1. Preheat oven to 375°F (190°C).
2. In a bowl, mix almond flour, Greek yogurt, eggs, baking powder, salt, and black pepper to form a dough. Spread the dough onto a parchment-lined baking sheet to form a thin crust.
3. Bake for 10 minutes until lightly golden.
4. Remove from oven and top with shredded mozzarella, crumbled bacon, cherry tomatoes, and chopped spinach. Drizzle with olive oil.
5. Return to oven and bake for an additional 10 minutes until cheese is melted and bubbly.

Nutritional Facts (Per Serving): Calories: 400 | Sugars: 4g | Fat: 27g | Carbohydrates: 18g | Protein: 20g | Fiber: 7g | Sodium: 600mg

Glycemic Index: Almond Flour: Low (GI = 15) | Greek Yogurt: Low (GI = 15) | Mozzarella Cheese: Low (GI = 34) | Bacon: Negligible GI (no carbs) | Cherry Tomatoes: Low (GI = 15) | Spinach: Low (GI = 15)

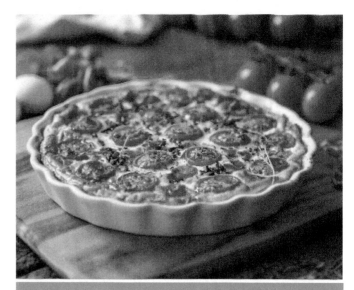

Turkey Bacon and Tomato Quiche

Prep: 15 mins | Cook: 30 mins | Serves: 2

Ingredients:

- 6 slices turkey bacon, cooked and crumbled (120g)
- 1 cup diced tomatoes (150g)
- 4 large eggs (200g)
- 1/2 cup almond flour (50g)
- 1/2 cup shredded mozzarella cheese (60g)
- 1/4 cup Greek yogurt (60g)
- 1/4 cup chopped spinach (30g)
- 1/4 tsp salt (1.5g)
- 1/4 tsp black pepper (1.5g)
- 1 tbsp olive oil (15ml)

Instructions:

1. Preheat oven to 375°F (190°C).
2. In a bowl, whisk eggs, Greek yogurt, almond flour, salt, and pepper.
3. Stir in cooked turkey bacon, diced tomatoes, mozzarella cheese, and chopped spinach.
4. Grease a baking dish with olive oil. Pour mixture into the dish and bake for 25-30 minutes until set and golden. Let cool slightly before serving.

Nutritional Facts (Per Serving): Calories: 400 | Sugars: 4g | Fat: 23g | Carbohydrates: 20g | Protein: 26g | Fiber: 7g | Sodium: 600mg

Glycemic Index: Turkey Bacon: Low (GI = 0) | Tomatoes: Low (GI = 15) | Eggs: Negligible GI (no carbs) | Almond Flour: Low (GI = 15) | Mozzarella Cheese: Low (GI = 34) | Greek Yogurt: Low (GI = 15) | Spinach: Low (GI = 15)

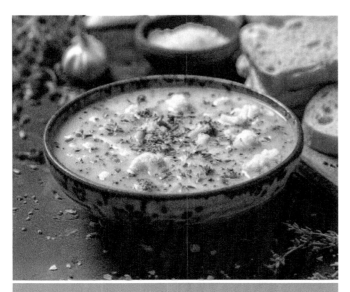

Cauliflower&Broccoli Cheese Soup

Prep: 10 mins | Cook: 30 mins | Serves: 2

Ingredients:

- 2 cups cauliflower florets (200g)
- 2 cups broccoli florets (200g)
- 4 cups low-sodium vegetable broth (960ml)
- 1 cup shredded cheddar cheese (100g)
- 1/2 cup heavy cream (120ml)
- 1 cup onion, chopped (150g)
- 2 cloves garlic, minced
- 1 tsp low carb sweeteners
- 1 tsp dried thyme (5g)
- Salt and pepper to taste

Instructions:

1. Sauté onions and garlic in a large pot until softened.
2. Add cauliflower, broccoli, and vegetable broth; bring to a boil. Simmer for 20 minutes until the vegetables are tender.
3. Stir in heavy cream, cheese, sweetener, and thyme; cook until the cheese melts and the soup is creamy. Season with salt and pepper to taste.

Nutritional Facts (Per Serving): Calories: 500 | Sugars: 5g | Fat: 22g | Carbohydrates: 55g | Protein: 25g | Fiber: 10g | Sodium: 780mg

Glycemic Index: Cauliflower: Low (GI = 15) | Broccoli: Low (GI = 15) | Cheese: Negligible GI | Cream: Negligible GI | Onion: Low (GI = 15) | Garlic: Low (GI = 15)

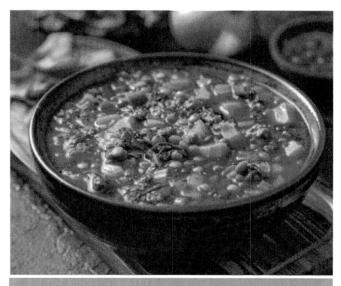

Hearty Lentil and Spinach Soup

Prep: 10 mins | Cook: 40 mins | Serves: 2

Ingredients:

- 1 cup dried lentils, rinsed (200g)
- 6 cups vegetable broth (1440ml)
- 1 cup diced tomatoes (240g)
- 2 cups fresh spinach, roughly chopped (60g)
- 3 cloves garlic, minced (9g)
- 1 medium onion, diced (150g)
- 2 medium carrots, diced (100g)
- 1 tbsp olive oil (15ml)
- 1 tsp ground cumin (2g)
- Salt and pepper, to taste

Instructions:

1. In a large pot, sauté onions, garlic, carrots, and celery over medium heat until softened, about 5 minutes.
2. Add lentils and vegetable broth. Bring to a boil. Reduce heat and simmer for 30 minutes until lentils are tender. Stir in spinach and cook for another 5 minutes.
3. Season with cumin, paprika, low carb sweeteners, salt, and pepper to taste.

Nutritional Facts (Per Serving): Calories: 500 | Sugars: 7g | Fat: 18g | Carbohydrates: 60g | Protein: 25g | Fiber: 10g | Sodium: 750mg

Glycemic Index: Lentils: Low (GI = 32) | Carrots: Low (GI = 39) | Celery: Low (GI = 15) | Onion: Low (GI = 15) | Spinach: Negligible GI

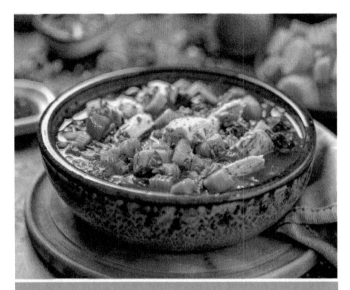

Chicken and Vegetable Stew

Prep: 15 mins | Cook: 45 mins | Serves: 2

Ingredients:

- 1 lb chicken breast, diced (450g)
- 2 cups low-sodium chicken broth (480ml)
- 1 cup carrots, sliced (120g)
- 1 cup celery, chopped (100g)
- 1 cup onion, chopped (150g)
- 2 cups spinach, chopped (60g)
- 1 tsp low carb sweeteners
- 1 tsp dried thyme (5g)
- 1 tsp dried rosemary (5g)
- Salt and pepper to taste

Instructions:

1. In a large pot, sauté onions, carrots, and celery over medium heat until softened, about 5 minutes.
2. Add chicken and cook until browned, about 8 minutes.
3. Pour in the chicken broth, add thyme and rosemary, and bring to a boil.
4. Reduce heat and simmer for 25 minutes.
5. Add spinach and cook for another 5 minutes until wilted.
6. Season with low carb sweeteners, salt, and pepper to taste.

Nutritional Facts (Per Serving): Calories: 500 | Sugars: 6g | Fat: 20g | Carbohydrates: 55g | Protein: 30g | Fiber: 9g | Sodium: 780mg

Glycemic Index: Chicken: Negligible GI | Carrots: Low (GI = 39) | Celery: Low (GI = 15) | Onion: Low (GI = 15) | Spinach: Negligible GI

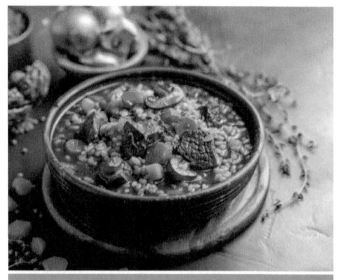

Beef and Barley Stew

Prep: 15 mins | Cook: 1 hour | Serves: 2

Ingredients:

- 1/2 lb beef stew meat, cubed (225g)
- 4 cups low-sodium beef broth (960ml)
- 1/2 cup pearl barley (100g)
- 1 cup carrots, diced (120g)
- 1 cup celery, chopped (100g)
- 1 cup onion, chopped (150g)
- 1 cup mushrooms, sliced (100g)
- 1 tsp dried thyme (5g)
- 1 tsp low carb sweeteners
- Salt and pepper to taste

Instructions:

1. In a large pot, brown the beef over medium heat until seared, about 5 minutes.
2. Add onions, carrots, celery, and mushrooms, and cook until softened, about 5 minutes.
3. Pour in the beef broth and add barley. Bring to a boil.
4. Reduce heat and simmer for 45 minutes, stirring occasionally.
5. Add thyme, low carb sweeteners, salt, and pepper. Cook for an additional 10 minutes.

Nutritional Facts (Per Serving): Calories: 500 | Sugars: 6g | Fat: 20g | Carbohydrates: 55g | Protein: 30g | Fiber: 10g | Sodium: 750mg

Glycemic Index: Beef: Negligible GI | Barley: Low (GI = 28) | Carrots: Low (GI = 39) | Celery: Low (GI = 15) | Onion: Low (GI = 15) | Mushrooms: Low (GI = 15)

CHAPTER 10: LUNCHES: Nutritious Grain And Legume Dishes

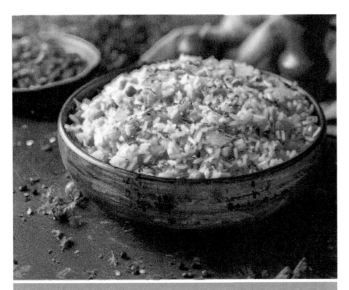

Brown Rice Pilaf

Prep: 10 mins | Cook: 40 mins | Serves: 2

Ingredients:

- 1 cup brown rice (185g)
- 2 cups low-sodium chicken broth (480ml)
- 1/2 cup carrots, diced (60g)
- 1/2 cup celery, diced (50g)
- 1/2 cup onion, chopped (75g)
- 1/4 cup peas (35g)
- 2 tbsp olive oil (30ml)
- 1 tsp dried thyme (5g)
- 1 tsp low carb sweeteners
- Salt and pepper to taste

Instructions:

1. Heat olive oil in a large pot over medium. Sauté onion, carrots, and celery for 5 minutes.
2. Add brown rice and cook, stirring, for 2 minutes.
3. Pour in chicken broth, add thyme, and boil.
4. Reduce heat to low, cover, and simmer for 35 minutes.
5. Stir in peas and cook for an additional 5 minutes.
6. Season with sweeteners, salt, and pepper.

Nutritional Facts (Per Serving): Calories: 500 | Sugars: 6g | Fat: 20g | Carbohydrates: 60g | Protein: 25g | Fiber: 10g | Sodium: 750mg

Glycemic Index: Brown Rice: Moderate (GI = 50) | Carrots: Low (GI = 39) | Celery: Low (GI = 15) | Peas: Low (GI = 22) | Onion: Low (GI = 15)

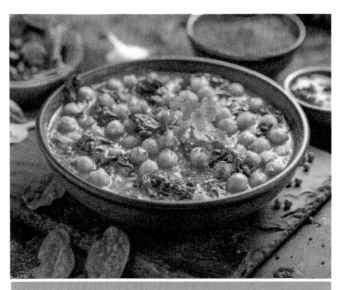

Chickpea and Spinach Curry

Prep: 10 mins | Cook: 30 mins | Serves: 2

Ingredients:

- 1 can chickpeas, drained and rinsed (15 oz/425g)
- 4 cups spinach, chopped (120g)
- 1 cup coconut milk (240ml)
- 1/2 cup onion, chopped (75g)
- 2 cloves garlic, minced
- 1 tbsp olive oil (15ml)
- 1 tsp curry powder (5g)
- 1 tsp cumin (5g)
- 1 tsp low carb sweeteners
- Salt and pepper to taste

Instructions:

1. Heat olive oil in a large pot over medium. Sauté onion and garlic for 5 minutes.
2. Stir in curry powder and cumin, and cook for 1 minute.
3. Add chickpeas, coconut milk, and spinach. Bring to a boil.
4. Reduce heat and simmer for 20 minutes.
5. Season with sweeteners, salt, and pepper.

Nutritional Facts (Per Serving): Calories: 500 | Sugars: 5g | Fat: 22g | Carbohydrates: 55g | Protein: 25g | Fiber: 10g | Sodium: 780mg

Glycemic Index: Chickpeas: Low (GI = 28) | Spinach: Negligible GI | Coconut Milk: Low (GI = 40) | Onion: Low (GI = 15) | Garlic: Low (GI = 15)

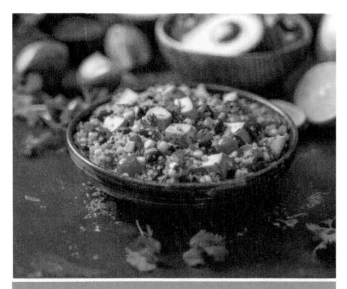

Quinoa and Black Bean Salad with Avocado

Prep: 15 mins | Cook: 15 mins | Serves: 2

Ingredients:

- 1/2 cup quinoa, rinsed (90g)
- 1 cup water (240ml)
- 1 cup black beans, drained and rinsed (240g)
- 1 avocado, diced (150g)
- 1 cup cherry tomatoes, halved (150g)
- 1/2 cup corn kernels (80g)
- 1/4 cup red onion, finely chopped (40g)
- 1/4 cup cilantro, chopped (15g)
- 2 tbsp lime juice (30ml)
- 1 tbsp olive oil (15ml)
- 1 tsp low carb sweeteners
- Salt and pepper to taste

Instructions:

1. Cook quinoa in water according to package instructions, about 15 minutes. Let cool.
2. In a large bowl, combine cooked quinoa, black beans, avocado, cherry tomatoes, corn, red onion, and cilantro.
3. In a small bowl, whisk together lime juice, olive oil, low carb sweeteners, salt, and pepper.
4. Pour the dressing over the salad and toss to combine.

Nutritional Facts (Per Serving): Calories: 500 | Sugars: 6g | Fat: 20g | Carbohydrates: 62g | Protein: 25g | Fiber: 10g | Sodium: 750mg

Glycemic Index: Quinoa: Low (GI = 53) | Black Beans: Low (GI = 30) | Avocado: Negligible GI | Tomatoes: Low (GI = 15) | Corn: Moderate (GI = 52)

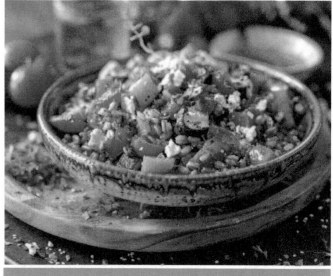

Farro and Roasted Vegetable Bowl

Prep: 20 mins | Cook: 30 mins | Serves: 2

Ingredients:

- 1/2 cup farro (90g)
- 1 cup water (240ml)
- 1 cup bell peppers, diced (150g)
- 1 cup zucchini, diced (150g)
- 1 cup cherry tomatoes, halved (150g)
- 1/2 cup red onion, chopped (75g)
- 2 tbsp olive oil (30ml)
- 1 tsp dried oregano (5g)
- 1 tsp low carb sweeteners
- Salt and pepper to taste
- 1/4 cup feta cheese, crumbled (30g)

Instructions:

1. Cook farro in water according to package instructions, about 20 minutes. Let cool.
2. Preheat oven to 400°F (200°C).
3. Toss bell peppers, zucchini, cherry tomatoes, and red onion with olive oil, oregano, low carb sweeteners, salt, and pepper.
4. Spread vegetables on a baking sheet and roast for 20 minutes until tender.
5. In a bowl, combine cooked farro and roasted vegetables. Top with crumbled feta cheese.

Nutritional Facts (Per Serving): Calories: 500 | Sugars: 7g | Fat: 22g | Carbohydrates: 60g | Protein: 25g | Fiber: 10g | Sodium: 800mg

Glycemic Index: Farro: Moderate (GI = 45) | Bell Peppers: Low (GI = 15) | Zucchini: Low (GI = 15) | Tomatoes: Low (GI = 15) | Red Onion: Low (GI = 15) | Feta Cheese: Low (GI = 15)

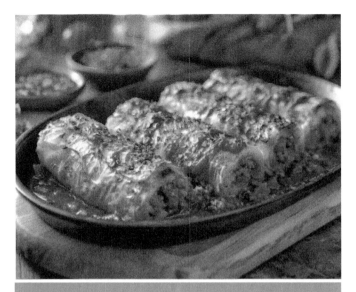

Stuffed Cabbage Rolls with Ground Turkey and Quinoa

Prep: 20 mins | Cook: 40 mins | Serves: 2

Ingredients:

- 4 large cabbage leaves (200g)
- 1/2 lb ground turkey (225g)
- 1/2 cup cooked quinoa (90g)
- 1/2 cup tomato sauce (120ml)
- 1/4 cup onion, chopped (35g)
- 1 clove garlic, minced
- 1 tsp dried oregano (5g)
- 1 tsp low carb sweeteners
- Salt and pepper to taste

Instructions:

1. Preheat oven to 375°F (190°C). Blanch cabbage leaves in boiling water for 2 minutes, then set aside.
2. In a large bowl, combine ground turkey, cooked quinoa, onion, garlic, oregano, low carb sweeteners, salt, and pepper.
3. Place a portion of the turkey mixture onto each cabbage leaf, roll up, and secure with toothpicks.
4. Place rolls in a baking dish, pour tomato sauce over the top, cover with foil, and bake for 35 minutes.

Nutritional Facts (Per Serving): Calories: 500 | Sugars: 7g | Fat: 18g | Carbohydrates: 55g | Protein: 30g | Fiber: 10g | Sodium: 750mg

Glycemic Index: Cabbage: Low (GI = 10) | Quinoa: Low (GI = 53) | Turkey: Negligible GI | Tomato Sauce: Low (GI = 15) | Onion: Low (GI = 15) | Garlic: Low (GI = 15)

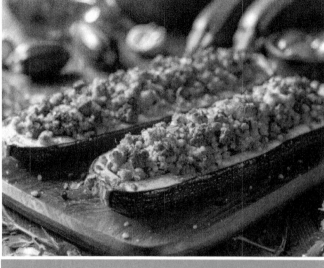

Zucchini Stuffed with Couscous and Meat

Prep: 15 mins | Cook: 30 mins | Serves: 2

Ingredients:

- 2 large zucchinis, halved lengthwise and seeded (400g)
- 1/2 cup couscous (90g)
- 1/2 cup low-sodium chicken broth (120ml)
- 1/2 lb ground beef (225g)
- 1/4 cup onion, chopped (35g)
- 1 clove garlic, minced
- 1/4 cup tomato sauce (60ml)
- 1 tsp dried basil (5g)
- 1 tsp low carb sweeteners
- Salt and pepper to taste

Instructions:

1. Preheat oven to 375°F (190°C). Place zucchinis cut-side up on a baking sheet.
2. Cook couscous in chicken broth according to package instructions, then set aside.
3. In a skillet, cook ground beef with onion and garlic until browned. Stir in cooked couscous, tomato sauce, basil, low carb sweeteners, salt, and pepper.
4. Spoon the mixture into the zucchini halves. Bake for 25 minutes until zucchinis are tender.

Nutritional Facts (Per Serving): Calories: 500 | Sugars: 6g | Fat: 20g | Carbohydrates: 60g | Protein: 25g | Fiber: 10g | Sodium: 780mg

Glycemic Index: Zucchini: Low (GI = 15) | Couscous: Moderate (GI = 65) | Beef: Negligible GI | Tomato Sauce: Low (GI = 15) | Onion: Low (GI = 15) | Garlic: Low (GI = 15)

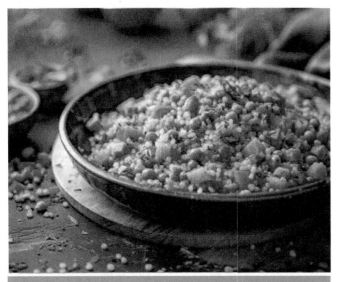

Green Buckwheat Pilaf

Prep: 10 mins | Cook: 30 mins | Serves: 2

Ingredients:

- 1 cup green buckwheat (180g)
- 2 cups water (480ml)
- 1/2 cup carrots, diced (60g)
- 1/2 cup bell pepper, diced (75g)
- 1/2 cup onion, chopped (75g)
- 1/4 cup peas (35g)
- 2 tbsp olive oil (30ml)
- 1 tsp dried thyme (5g)
- 1 tsp low carb sweeteners
- Salt and pepper to taste

Instructions:

1. Heat olive oil in a large pot over medium heat. Add onion, carrots, and bell pepper, and sauté until softened, about 5 minutes.
2. Add green buckwheat and cook, stirring, for 2 minutes. Pour in water, add thyme, and bring to a boil.
3. Reduce heat to low, cover, and simmer for 20 minutes. Stir in peas and cook for an additional 5 minutes.
4ю. Season with low carb sweeteners, salt, and pepper to taste.

Nutritional Facts (Per Serving): Calories: 500 | Sugars: 5g | Fat: 20g | Carbohydrates: 60g | Protein: 25g | Fiber: 10g | Sodium: 750mg

Glycemic Index: Green Buckwheat: Low (GI = 50) | Carrots: Low (GI = 39) | Bell Pepper: Low (GI = 15) | Peas: Low (GI = 22) | Onion: Low (GI = 15)

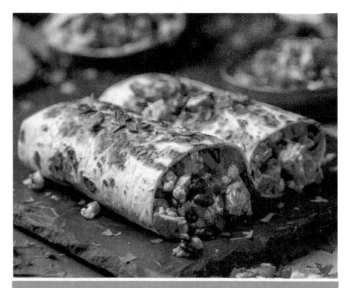

Wild Rice with Cauliflower and Chicken Burrito

Prep: 15 mins | Cook: 30 mins | Serves: 2

Ingredients:

- 1 cup low-sodium chicken broth (240ml)
- 1 cup cauliflower, chopped (100g)
- 1/2 lb chicken breast, diced (225g)
- 1/2 cup bell pepper, diced (75g)
- 1/2 cup onion, chopped (75g)
- 1/4 cup black beans, drained and rinsed (60g)
- 2 tbsp olive oil (30ml)
- 1 tsp cumin (5g)
- 1 tsp low carb sweeteners
- Salt and pepper to taste
- 2 whole-wheat tortillas (60g each)
- 1/2 cup wild rice (85g)

Instructions:

1. Cook wild rice in chicken broth according to package instructions; let cool.
2. Sauté onion, bell pepper, and cauliflower in olive oil over medium heat until softened.
3. Add diced chicken to the skillet and cook until browned.
4. Stir in black beans, cooked wild rice, cumin, sweetener, salt, and pepper; cook for 5 more minutes.
5. Assemble burritos by spooning the mixture onto tortillas and wrapping them up.

Nutritional Facts (Per Serving): Calories: 500 | Sugars: 6g | Fat: 22g | Carbohydrates: 60g | Protein: 25g | Fiber: 10g | Sodium: 780mg

Glycemic Index: Wild Rice: Moderate (GI = 45) | Cauliflower: Low (GI = 15) | Chicken: Negligible GI | Bell Pepper: Low (GI = 15) | Black Beans: Low (GI = 30) | Whole-Wheat Tortilla: Moderate (GI = 50)

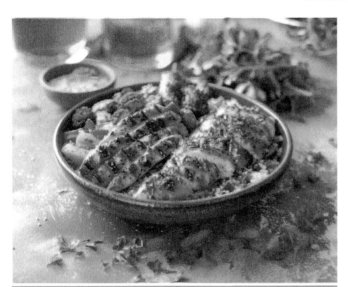

Grilled Chicken and Veggie Bowl

Prep: 15 mins | Cook: 20 mins | Serves: 2

Ingredients:

- 2 chicken breasts (300g)
- 1 cup broccoli florets (150g)
- 1 cup bell peppers, sliced (150g)
- 1 cup zucchini, sliced (150g)
- 2 tbsp olive oil (30ml)
- 1 tbsp lemon juice (15ml)
- 1 tsp dried oregano (5g)
- 1 tsp low carb sweeteners
- Salt and pepper to taste
- 1/2 cup quinoa, cooked (90g)

Instructions:

1. Preheat grill to medium heat.
2. Marinate chicken breasts in lemon juice, 1 tbsp olive oil, oregano, salt, and pepper for 10 minutes.
3. Grill chicken for 6-7 minutes per side until fully cooked. Toss broccoli, bell peppers, and zucchini in remaining olive oil, salt, and pepper.
4. Grill vegetables until tender, about 5-7 minutes.
5. Slice grilled chicken and serve over cooked quinoa with grilled vegetables.

Nutritional Facts (Per Serving): Calories: 500 | Sugars: 5g | Fat: 20g | Carbohydrates: 55g | Protein: 30g | Fiber: 10g | Sodium: 750mg

Glycemic Index: Chicken: Negligible GI | Broccoli: Low (GI = 15) | Bell Peppers: Low (GI = 15) | Zucchini: Low (GI = 15) | Quinoa: Low (GI = 53)

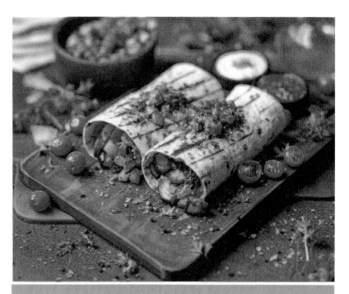

Roasted Veggie and Hummus Wrap

Prep: 10 mins | Cook: 25 mins | Serves: 2

Ingredients:

- 1 cup eggplant, diced (150g)
- 1 cup zucchini, diced (150g)
- 1 cup bell peppers, diced (150g)
- 1/2 cup cherry tomatoes, halved (75g)
- 2 tbsp olive oil (30ml)
- 1 tsp dried basil (5g)
- 1 tsp low carb sweeteners
- Salt and pepper to taste
- 1/2 cup hummus (120g)
- 2 whole-wheat tortillas (60g each)

Instructions:

1. Preheat oven to 400°F (200°C).
2. Toss eggplant, zucchini, bell peppers, and cherry tomatoes in olive oil, basil, low carb sweeteners, salt, and pepper.
3. Spread vegetables on a baking sheet and roast for 20 minutes until tender.
4. Spread hummus evenly on each tortilla.
5. Add roasted vegetables and wrap the tortillas.

Nutritional Facts (Per Serving): Calories: 500 | Sugars: 6g | Fat: 20g | Carbohydrates: 60g | Protein: 25g | Fiber: 10g | Sodium: 780mg

Glycemic Index: Eggplant: Low (GI = 15) | Zucchini: Low (GI = 15) | Bell Peppers: Low (GI = 15) | Cherry Tomatoes: Low (GI = 15) | Hummus: Low (GI = 15) | Whole-Wheat Tortilla: Moderate (GI = 50)

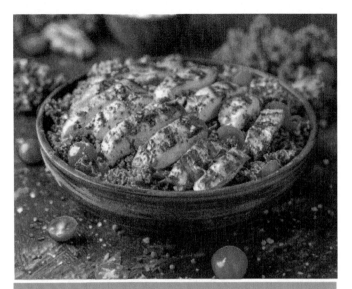

Kale and Chicken Caesar Salad

Prep: 15 mins | Cook: 15 mins | Serves: 2

Ingredients:

- 2 chicken breasts, grilled and sliced (300g)
- 4 cups kale, chopped (120g)
- 1/2 cup Caesar dressing (120ml)
- 1/4 cup grated Parmesan cheese (30g)
- 1/2 cup cherry tomatoes, halved (75g)
- 2 tbsp olive oil (30ml)
- 1 tsp low carb sweeteners
- Salt and pepper to taste

Instructions:

1. Massage kale with 1 tbsp olive oil and a pinch of salt until tender.
2. In a large bowl, combine kale, cherry tomatoes, and Parmesan cheese.
3. While preparing the kale, grill the chicken breasts until they are thoroughly cooked and have clear grill marks, about 6-7 minutes on each side. Allow the chicken to rest for a few minutes, then slice.
4. Add grilled chicken slices and toss with Caesar dressing.
5. Season with low carb sweeteners, salt, and pepper to taste.

Nutritional Facts (Per Serving): Calories: 500 | Sugars: 6g | Fat: 22g | Carbohydrates: 50g | Protein: 30g | Fiber: 8g | Sodium: 750mg

Glycemic Index: Kale: Low (GI = 15) | Chicken: Negligible GI | Caesar Dressing: Low (GI = 30) | Parmesan Cheese: Low (GI = 15) | Cherry Tomatoes: Low (GI = 15)

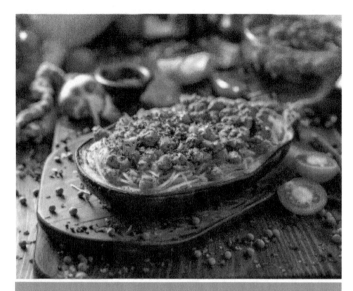

Spaghetti Squash with Turkey Marinara

Prep: 15 mins | Cook: 40 mins | Serves: 2

Ingredients:

- 1 medium spaghetti squash (800g)
- 1/2 lb ground turkey (225g)
- 2 cups tomato sauce (480ml)
- 1/2 cup onion, chopped (75g)
- 1/2 cup bell peppers, diced (75g)
- 2 cloves garlic, minced
- 2 tbsp olive oil (30ml)
- 1 tsp dried basil (5g)
- 1 tsp low carb sweeteners
- Salt and pepper to taste

Instructions:

1. Preheat oven to 400°F (200°C). Cut spaghetti squash in half, remove seeds, and brush with 1 tbsp olive oil. Place cut-side down on a baking sheet and roast for 35 minutes.
2. In a skillet, heat remaining olive oil over medium heat. Add onion, bell peppers, and garlic, and sauté until softened, about 5 minutes.
3. Add ground turkey and cook until browned.
4. Stir in tomato sauce, basil, low carb sweeteners, salt, and pepper. Simmer for 10 minutes.
5. Scrape out the spaghetti squash strands with a fork and place in a bowl. Top with turkey marinara.

Nutritional Facts (Per Serving): Calories: 500 | Sugars: 7g | Fat: 20g | Carbohydrates: 60g | Protein: 25g | Fiber: 10g | Sodium: 780mg

Glycemic Index: Spaghetti Squash: Low (GI = 20) | Turkey: Negligible GI | Tomato Sauce: Low (GI = 15) | Onion: Low (GI = 15) | Bell Peppers: Low (GI = 15)

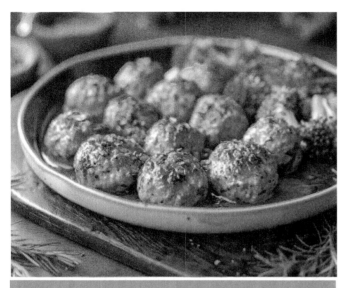

Broccoli and Turkey Meatball Lunch Box

Prep: 15 mins | Cook: 20 mins | Serves: 2

Ingredients:

- 1/2 lb ground turkey (225g)
- 1/2 cup breadcrumbs (60g)
- 1/4 cup Parmesan cheese, grated (30g)
- 1 egg (50g)
- 1 tsp dried oregano (5g)
- 1 tsp low carb sweeteners
- Salt and pepper to taste
- 2 cups broccoli florets (300g)
- 1 tbsp olive oil (15ml)

Instructions:

1. Preheat oven to 375°F (190°C). Mix ground turkey, breadcrumbs, Parmesan, egg, oregano, sweeteners, salt, and pepper in a bowl. Form into meatballs and arrange on a baking sheet. Bake for 20 minutes.
2. Steam broccoli until tender, about 5-7 minutes, then drizzle with olive oil.
3. Place meatballs and broccoli in lunch boxes.

Nutritional Facts (Per Serving): Calories: 500 | Sugars: 4g | Fat: 20g | Carbohydrates: 50g | Protein: 30g | Fiber: 8g | Sodium: 750mg

Glycemic Index: Turkey: Negligible GI | Breadcrumbs: Moderate (GI = 70) | Parmesan Cheese: Low (GI = 15) | Broccoli: Low (GI = 15)

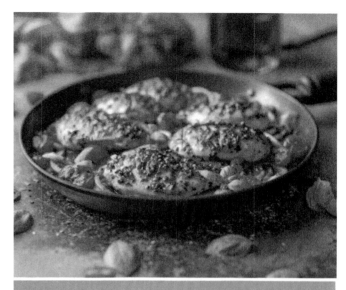

Zucchini Noodles with Pesto Chicken

Prep: 15 mins | Cook: 20 mins | Serves: 2

Ingredients:

- 2 chicken breasts, sliced (300g)
- 4 cups zucchini noodles (400g)
- 1/4 cup basil pesto (60g)
- 1/2 cup cherry tomatoes, halved (75g)
- 1/4 cup Parmesan cheese, grated (30g)
- 2 tbsp olive oil (30ml)
- 1 tsp low carb sweeteners
- Salt and pepper to taste

Instructions:

1. In a skillet, heat 1 tbsp olive oil over medium heat. Add chicken slices, season with salt and pepper, and cook until browned and cooked through, about 6-7 minutes.
2. Remove chicken from skillet and set aside. In the same skillet, add remaining olive oil and zucchini noodles. Sauté for 3-4 minutes until tender.
3. Return chicken to the skillet, add pesto, and cherry tomatoes. Toss to combine and heat through for 2-3 minutes.
4. Sprinkle with Parmesan cheese before serving.

Nutritional Facts (Per Serving): Calories: 500 | Sugars: 5g | Fat: 22g | Carbohydrates: 50g | Protein: 30g | Fiber: 10g | Sodium: 780mg

Glycemic Index: Chicken: Negligible GI | Zucchini: Low (GI = 15) | Pesto: Low (GI = 15) | Cherry Tomatoes: Low (GI = 15) | Parmesan Cheese: Low (GI = 15)

CHAPTER 12: LUNCHES: Protein-rich Lunch Ideas

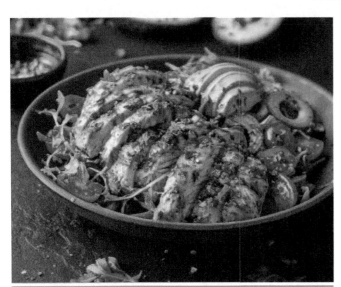

Chicken and Avocado Salad

Prep: 15 mins | Cook: 10 mins | Serves: 2

Ingredients:

- 2 chicken breasts, grilled and sliced (300g)
- 1 avocado, diced (150g)
- 4 cups mixed greens (120g)
- 1/2 cup cherry tomatoes, halved (75g)
- 1/4 cup red onion, thinly sliced (35g)
- 2 tbsp olive oil (30ml)
- 1 tbsp lemon juice (15ml)
- 1 tsp low carb sweeteners
- Salt and pepper to taste

Instructions:

1. In a large bowl, combine mixed greens, cherry tomatoes, red onion, and avocado.
2. In a small bowl, whisk together olive oil, lemon juice, low carb sweeteners, salt, and pepper.
3. Add grilled chicken slices to the salad and drizzle with the dressing. Toss to combine.

Nutritional Facts (Per Serving): Calories: 500 | Sugars: 5g | Fat: 22g | Carbohydrates: 50g | Protein: 30g | Fiber: 10g | Sodium: 750mg

Glycemic Index: Chicken: Negligible GI | Avocado: Negligible GI | Mixed Greens: Low (GI = 15) | Cherry Tomatoes: Low (GI = 15) | Red Onion: Low (GI = 15)

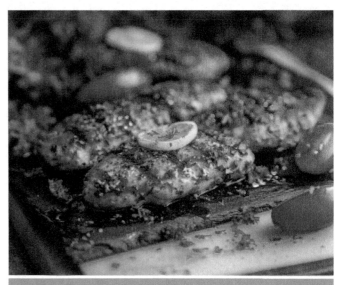

Chicken and Turkey Cutlets

Prep: 15 mins | Cook: 20 mins | Serves: 2

Ingredients:

- 1/2 lb ground chicken (225g)
- 1/2 lb ground turkey (225g)
- 2 hard-boiled eggs, chopped (100g)
- 1/4 cup breadcrumbs (30g)
- 1 tsp low carb sweeteners
- 1 clove garlic, minced
- 1/4 cup onion, finely chopped (35g)
- 1 tbsp olive oil (15ml)
- Salt and pepper to taste

Instructions:

1. In a large bowl, combine ground chicken, ground turkey, chopped hard-boiled eggs, breadcrumbs, onion, garlic, low carb sweeteners, salt, and pepper. Mix well. Form the mixture into cutlets.
3. Heat olive oil in a frying pan over medium heat. Fry cutlets until golden brown and cooked through, about 6-7 minutes per side.

Nutritional Facts (Per Serving): Calories: 500 | Sugars: 4g | Fat: 20g | Carbohydrates: 50g | Protein: 30g | Fiber: 8g | Sodium: 780mg

Glycemic Index: Chicken: Negligible GI | Turkey: Negligible GI | Hard-boiled Eggs: Negligible GI | Breadcrumbs: Moderate (GI = 70) | Onion: Low (GI = 15) | Garlic: Low (GI = 15)

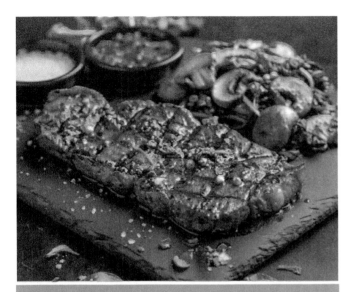

Seared Ribeye Steak with Sautéed Spinach and Mushrooms

Prep: 10 mins | Cook: 15 mins | Serves: 2

Ingredients:

- 2 ribeye steaks (300g each)
- 2 tbsp olive oil (30ml)
- 2 cups spinach (60g)
- 1 cup mushrooms, sliced (100g)
- 2 cloves garlic, minced
- 1 tsp low carb sweeteners
- Salt and pepper to taste

Instructions:

1. Heat 1 tbsp olive oil in a skillet over medium-high heat. Season steaks with salt and pepper, and sear for 3-4 minutes per side for medium-rare. Remove and let rest.
2. In the same skillet, add remaining olive oil and garlic. Sauté for 1 minute.
3. Add mushrooms and cook until tender, about 5 minutes.
4. Add spinach and cook until wilted, about 2 minutes. Serve steaks with sautéed spinach and mushrooms.

Nutritional Facts (Per Serving): Calories: 500 | Sugars: 2g | Fat: 22g | Carbohydrates: 50g | Protein: 30g | Fiber: 8g | Sodium: 700mg

Glycemic Index: Ribeye Steak: Negligible GI | Spinach: Low (GI = 15) | Mushrooms: Low (GI = 15) | Garlic: Low (GI = 15)

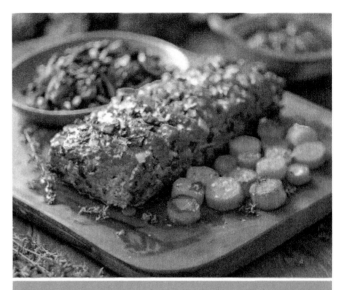

Turkey Meatloaf with Spinach and Roasted Vegetables

Prep: 15 mins | Cook: 45 mins | Serves: 2

Ingredients:

- 1 lb ground turkey (450g)
- 1 cup spinach, chopped (30g)
- 1/2 cup breadcrumbs (60g)
- 1 egg (50g)
- 1/4 cup onion, chopped (35g)
- 1 clove garlic, minced
- 1 tsp dried oregano (5g)
- 1 tsp low carb sweeteners
- Salt and pepper to taste
- 1 cup carrots, sliced (120g)
- 1 cup bell peppers, sliced (150g)
- 2 tbsp olive oil (30ml)

Instructions:

1. Preheat oven to 375°F (190°C). In a bowl, combine ground turkey, spinach, breadcrumbs, egg, onion, garlic, oregano, low carb sweeteners, salt, and pepper. Mix well and shape into a loaf.
2. Place meatloaf in a baking dish. Toss carrots and bell peppers with olive oil, salt, and pepper, and arrange around the meatloaf.
3. Bake for 45 minutes until meatloaf is cooked through and vegetables are tender.

Nutritional Facts (Per Serving): Calories: 500 | Sugars: 7g | Fat: 20g | Carbohydrates: 50g | Protein: 30g | Fiber: 10g | Sodium: 750mg

Glycemic Index: Turkey: Negligible GI | Spinach: Low (GI = 15) | Breadcrumbs: Moderate (GI = 70) | Carrots: Low (GI = 39) | Bell Peppers: Low (GI = 15)

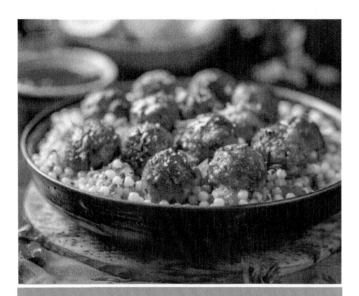

Meatballs with Couscous

Prep: 15 mins | Cook: 30 mins | Serves: 2

Ingredients:

- 1/2 lb ground turkey (225g)
- 1/2 cup couscous (90g)
- 1 egg (50g)
- 1/4 cup onion, finely chopped (35g)
- 1 clove garlic, minced
- 1/2 cup sour cream (120ml)
- 1 cup chicken broth (240ml)
- 1 tbsp olive oil (15ml)
- 1 tsp dried thyme (5g)
- 1 tsp low carb sweeteners
- Salt and pepper to taste

Instructions:

1. Preheat oven to 375°F (190°C). Cook couscous according to package instructions and let cool.
2. In a bowl, combine ground turkey, cooked couscous, egg, onion, garlic, thyme, low carb sweeteners, salt, and pepper. Mix well and shape into meatballs.
3. Heat olive oil in a skillet. Brown meatballs then transfer to a baking dish. In a bowl, mix sour cream and chicken broth. Pour over meatballs.
4. Bake for 20 minutes.

Nutritional Facts (Per Serving): Calories: 500 | Sugars: 5g | Fat: 20g | Carbohydrates: 55g | Protein: 30g | Fiber: 8g | Sodium: 780mg

Glycemic Index: Turkey: Negligible GI | Couscous: Moderate (GI = 65) | Sour Cream: Low (GI = 30) | Onion: Low (GI = 15) | Garlic: Low (GI = 15)

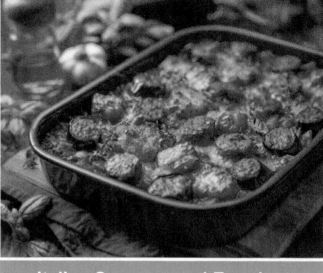

Italian Sausage and Eggplant Casserole

Prep: 15 mins | Cook: 40 mins | Serves: 2

Ingredients:

- 1/2 lb Italian sausage, sliced (225g)
- 1 large eggplant, diced (400g)
- 1 cup tomato sauce (240ml)
- 1/2 cup mozzarella cheese, shredded (60g)
- 1/2 cup onion, chopped (75g)
- 2 cloves garlic, minced
- 2 tbsp olive oil (30ml)
- 1 tsp dried oregano (5g)
- 1 tsp low carb sweeteners
- Salt and pepper to taste
- 1/4 cup Parmesan cheese, grated (30g)

Instructions:

1. Preheat oven to 375°F (190°C). Cook sausage in 1 tbsp olive oil over medium heat until browned.
2. In the same skillet, sauté onion and garlic in remaining olive oil until softened.
3. Add diced eggplant and cook until tender. Stir in tomato sauce, oregano, sweetener, salt, and pepper; cook for 5 minutes.
4. Transfer mixture to a baking dish. Top with cooked sausage, mozzarella, and Parmesan cheese. Bake for 20 minutes.

Nutritional Facts (Per Serving): Calories: 500 | Sugars: 7g | Fat: 22g | Carbohydrates: 50g | Protein: 30g | Fiber: 10g | Sodium: 780mg

Glycemic Index: Italian Sausage: Negligible GI | Eggplant: Low (GI = 15) | Tomato Sauce: Low (GI = 15) | Mozzarella Cheese: Low (GI = 15) | Parmesan Cheese: Low (GI = 15) | Onion: Low (GI = 15) | Garlic: Low (GI = 15)

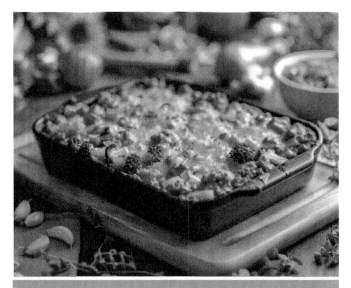

Ground Turkey and Vegetable Casserole

Prep: 15 mins | Cook: 40 mins | Serves: 2

Ingredients:

- 1 lb ground turkey (450g)
- 1 cup broccoli florets (150g)
- 1 cup bell peppers, diced (150g)
- 1/2 cup carrots, sliced (60g)
- 1/2 cup onion, chopped (75g)
- 1 cup low-sodium chicken broth (240ml)
- 1/2 cup shredded cheddar cheese (60g)
- 2 cloves garlic, minced
- 2 tbsp olive oil (30ml)
- 1 tsp dried thyme (5g)
- 1 tsp low carb sweeteners
- Salt and pepper to taste

Instructions:

1. Preheat oven to 375°F (190°C). Sauté garlic and onion in olive oil over medium heat until softened.
2. Add ground turkey and cook until browned.
3. Stir in broccoli, bell peppers, carrots, thyme, sweetener, salt, and pepper; cook for 5 minutes.
4. Pour in chicken broth and transfer the mixture to a baking dish. Top with shredded cheddar cheese.
5. Bake for 20 minutes until the cheese is melted and bubbly.

Nutritional Facts (Per Serving): Calories: 500 | Sugars: 6g | Fat: 20g | Carbohydrates: 55g | Protein: 30g | Fiber: 10g | Sodium: 780mg

Glycemic Index: Ground Turkey: Negligible GI | Broccoli: Low (GI = 15) | Bell Peppers: Low (GI = 15) | Carrots: Low (GI = 39) | Onion: Low (GI = 15) | Cheddar Cheese: Low (GI = 15)

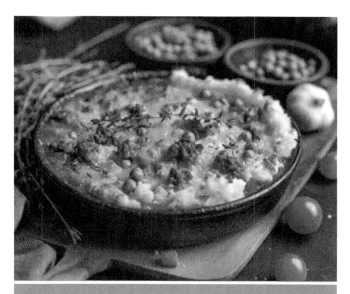

Cauliflower Shepherd's Pie

Prep: 20 mins | Cook: 40 mins | Serves: 2

Ingredients:

- 1/2 lb ground beef (225g)
- 2 cups cauliflower florets (300g)
-
- 1/2 cup carrots, diced (60g)
- 1/2 cup onion, chopped (75g)
- 1/4 cup low-sodium beef broth (60ml)
- 1/4 cup shredded cheddar cheese (30g)
- 2 cloves garlic, minced
- 2 tbsp olive oil (30ml)
- 1 tsp dried rosemary (5g)
- 1 tsp low carb sweeteners
- Salt and pepper to taste
- 1/2 cup peas (75g)

Instructions:

1. Preheat oven to 375°F (190°C). Steam cauliflower until tender, then mash and set aside.
2. Sauté garlic and onion in olive oil over medium heat until softened.
3. Add ground beef and cook until browned.
4. Stir in peas, carrots, rosemary, sweetener, salt, and pepper; cook for 5 minutes. Pour in beef broth and transfer the mixture to a baking dish.
5. Top with mashed cauliflower and sprinkle with cheddar cheese. Bake for 20 minutes until the cheese is melted and bubbly.

Nutritional Facts (Per Serving): Calories: 500 | Sugars: 6g | Fat: 20g | Carbohydrates: 55g | Protein: 30g | Fiber: 10g | Sodium: 750mg

Glycemic Index: Ground Beef: Negligible GI | Cauliflower: Low (GI = 15) | Peas: Low (GI = 22) | Carrots: Low (GI = 39) | Onion: Low (GI = 15) | Cheddar Cheese: Low (GI = 15)

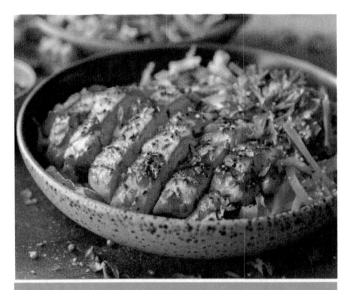

Fried Cabbage with Chicken

Prep: 10 mins | Cook: 20 mins | Serves: 2

Ingredients:

- 1/2 lb chicken fillet, cut into pieces (225g)
- 2 cups cabbage, shredded (300g)
- 1 cup onion, chopped (150g)
- 1 cup carrot, julienned (120g)
- 2 tbsp olive oil (30ml)
- 1 tsp low carb sweeteners
- Salt and pepper to taste

Instructions:

1. Heat 1 tbsp olive oil in a large skillet over medium heat. Add chicken pieces, season with salt and pepper, and cook until browned and cooked through, about 7-8 minutes. Remove and set aside.
2. In the same skillet, add remaining olive oil, onion, and carrot. Sauté until softened, about 5 minutes.
3. Add cabbage and cook until tender, about 7 minutes.
4. Return chicken to the skillet, add low carb sweeteners, salt, and pepper. Toss to combine and heat through.

Nutritional Facts (Per Serving):
Calories: 500 | Sugars: 6g | Fat: 20g | Carbohydrates: 55g | Protein: 30g | Fiber: 10g | Sodium: 750mg

Glycemic Index: Chicken: Negligible GI | Cabbage: Low (GI = 10) | Onion: Low (GI = 15) | Carrot: Low (GI = 39)

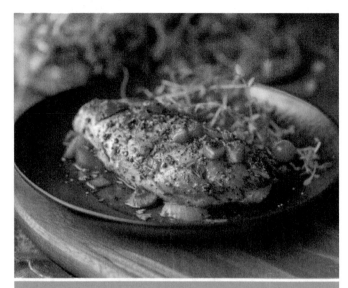

Chicken Stuffed with Buckwheat

Prep: 15 mins | Cook: 45 mins | Serves: 2

Ingredients:

- 2 chicken breasts (300g each)
- 1/2 cup buckwheat, cooked (90g)
- 1/4 cup mushrooms, chopped (35g)
- 1/4 cup onion, finely chopped (35g)
- 1 clove garlic, minced
- 2 tbsp olive oil (30ml)
- 1 tsp dried thyme (5g)
- 1 tsp low carb sweeteners
- Salt and pepper to taste

Instructions:

1. Preheat oven to 375°F (190°C). In a skillet, heat 1 tbsp olive oil over medium heat. Add onion, garlic, and mushrooms. Sauté until softened, about 5 minutes.
2. In a bowl, combine cooked buckwheat, sautéed vegetables, thyme, low carb sweeteners, salt, and pepper.
3. Cut a pocket into each chicken breast and stuff with the buckwheat mixture.
4. Heat remaining olive oil in a skillet over medium heat. Sear stuffed chicken breasts for 2-3 minutes per side until browned.
5. Transfer to a baking dish and bake for 25-30 minutes until chicken is cooked through.

Nutritional Facts (Per Serving): Calories: 500 | Sugars: 5g | Fat: 22g | Carbohydrates: 50g | Protein: 30g | Fiber: 10g | Sodium: 780mg

Glycemic Index: Chicken: Negligible GI | Buckwheat: Low (GI = 55) | Mushrooms: Low (GI = 15) | Onion: Low (GI = 15) | Garlic: Low (GI = 15)

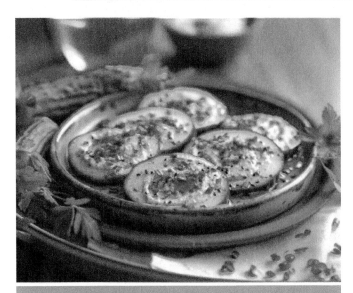

Cucumber Slices with Hummus

Prep: 10 mins | Cook: 0 mins | Serves: 2

Ingredients:

- 1 large cucumber (300g), sliced
- 1 cup hummus (250g)
- 1 tsp olive oil (5ml)
- 1 tsp lemon juice (5ml)
- 1/4 tsp paprika (1g)
- Salt to taste (1g)

Instructions:

1. Arrange cucumber slices on a serving plate.
2. In a small bowl, mix hummus with olive oil, lemon juice, and a pinch of salt.
3. Sprinkle paprika over the hummus.
4. Serve the hummus with cucumber slices.

Nutritional Facts (Per Serving): Calories: 250 | Sugars: 3g | Fat: 9g | Carbohydrates: 29g | Protein: 13g | Fiber: 5g | Sodium: 400mg

Glycemic Index: Cucumber: Low (GI = 15) | Hummus: Low (GI = 15) | Olive oil, lemon juice, paprika: Negligible GI

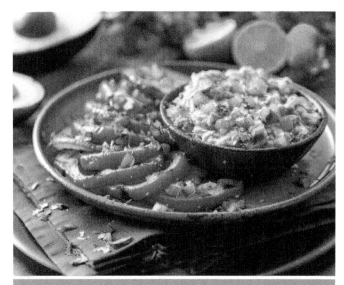

Sliced Bell Peppers with Guacamole

Prep: 10 mins | Cook: 0 mins | Serves: 2

Ingredients:

- 1 large bell pepper (200g), sliced
- 1 avocado (200g)
- 1/4 cup diced red onion (40g)
- 1 tbsp lime juice (15ml)
- 1 tbsp chopped cilantro (5g)
- 1/4 tsp salt (1g)
- 1/4 tsp cumin (1g)
- 1/4 tsp garlic powder (1g)

Instructions:

1. In a bowl, mash the avocado.
2. Add diced red onion, lime juice, chopped cilantro, salt, cumin, and garlic powder. Mix well.
3. Serve the guacamole with bell pepper slices.

Nutritional Facts (Per Serving): Calories: 250 | Sugars: 3g | Fat: 11g | Carbohydrates: 25g | Protein: 12g | Fiber: 5g | Sodium: 400mg

Glycemic Index: Bell pepper: Low (GI = 15) | Guacamole: Low (GI = 15)

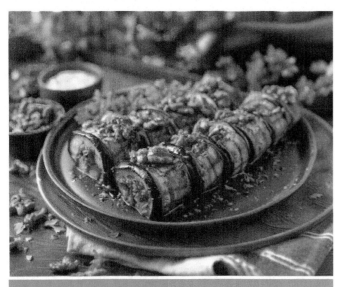

Eggplant Rolls with Nut Stuffing

Prep: 20 mins | Cook: 15 mins | Serves: 2

Ingredients:

- 1 large eggplant (300g), sliced lengthwise
- 1/2 cup walnuts (60g), finely chopped
- 1 tbsp olive oil (15ml)
- 1 tbsp lemon juice (15ml)
- 1 garlic clove, minced (5g)
- 2 tbsp parsley (10g), chopped
- Salt and pepper to taste (2g)

Instructions:

1. Preheat the oven to 375°F (190°C).
2. Brush eggplant slices with olive oil and season with salt and pepper.
3. Bake eggplant slices for 10 minutes until tender.
4. In a bowl, combine chopped walnuts, lemon juice, minced garlic, and chopped parsley.
5. Spread the walnut mixture on each eggplant slice and roll up.
6. Secure with toothpicks if necessary and serve.

Nutritional Facts (Per Serving): Calories: 250 | Sugars: 3g | Fat: 11g | Carbohydrates: 25g | Protein: 13g | Fiber: 5g | Sodium: 400mg

Glycemic Index: Eggplant: Low (GI = 15) | Walnuts: Low (GI = 15) | Olive oil, lemon juice, garlic, parsley: Negligible GI

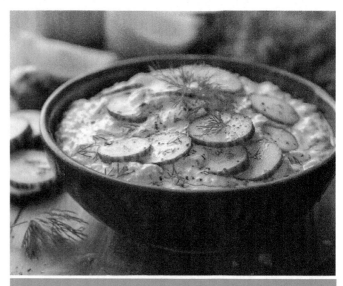

Greek Yogurt with Cucumbers

Prep: 10 mins | Cook: 0 mins | Serves: 2

Ingredients:

- 1 cup Greek yogurt (240g)
- 1 large cucumber (300g), diced
- 1 tbsp olive oil (15ml)
- 1 tbsp lemon juice (15ml)
- 1 garlic clove, minced (5g)
- 1 tbsp dill (5g), chopped
- Salt and pepper to taste (2g)

Instructions:

1. In a bowl, mix Greek yogurt with olive oil, lemon juice, and minced garlic.
2. Add diced cucumber and chopped dill, stirring to combine.
3. Season with salt and pepper to taste.
4. Serve chilled.

Nutritional Facts (Per Serving): Calories: 250 | Sugars: 4g | Fat: 9g | Carbohydrates: 27g | Protein: 15g | Fiber: 5g | Sodium: 400mg

Glycemic Index: Greek yogurt: Low (GI = 15) | Cucumber: Low (GI = 15) | Olive oil, lemon juice, garlic, dill: Negligible GI

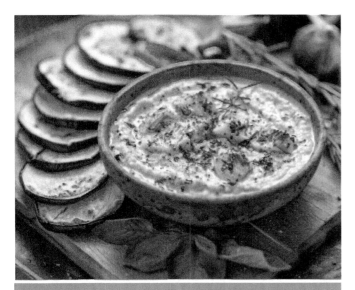

Artichoke and Spinach Yogurt Dip with Roasted Eggplant

Prep: 15 mins | Cook: 20 mins | Serves: 2

Ingredients:

- 1 cup Greek yogurt (240g)
- 1/2 cup artichoke hearts, chopped (120g)
- 1/2 cup fresh spinach, chopped (30g)
- 1/4 cup grated Parmesan cheese (25g)
- 1 garlic clove, minced (5g)
- 1 tbsp olive oil (15ml)
- 1 large eggplant (300g), sliced
- Salt and pepper to taste (2g)

Instructions:

1. Preheat oven to 400°F (200°C).
2. Brush eggplant slices with olive oil, season with salt and pepper, and roast for 15 minutes.
3. In a bowl, mix Greek yogurt, chopped artichoke hearts, chopped spinach, grated Parmesan, minced garlic, salt, and pepper.
4. Serve the dip with roasted eggplant slices.

Nutritional Facts (Per Serving): Calories: 250 | Sugars: 3g | Fat: 9g | Carbohydrates: 28g | Protein: 14g | Fiber: 5g | Sodium: 400mg

Glycemic Index: Greek yogurt: Low (GI = 15) | Artichoke hearts: Low (GI = 15) | Spinach: Low (GI = 15) | Eggplant: Low (GI = 15) | Parmesan, olive oil, garlic: Negligible GI

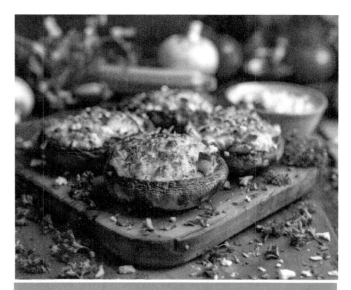

Zucchini and Feta Stuffed Mushrooms

Prep: 15 mins | Cook: 20 mins | Serves: 2

Ingredients:

- 8 large mushrooms (200g), stems removed
- 1 small zucchini, finely diced (150g)
- 1/2 cup feta cheese, crumbled (100g)
- 1 garlic clove, minced (5g)
- 1 tbsp olive oil (15ml)
- 1 tbsp chopped parsley (5g)
- Salt and pepper to taste (2g)

Instructions:

1. Preheat oven to 375°F (190°C).
2. In a bowl, mix diced zucchini, crumbled feta, minced garlic, chopped parsley, salt, and pepper.
3. Stuff each mushroom cap with the zucchini mixture.
4. Place stuffed mushrooms on a baking sheet, drizzle with olive oil, and bake for 20 minutes until mushrooms are tender.

Nutritional Facts (Per Serving): Calories: 250 | Sugars: 3g | Fat: 10g | Carbohydrates: 26g | Protein: 13g | Fiber: 4g | Sodium: 400mg

Glycemic Index: Mushrooms: Low (GI = 15) | Zucchini: Low (GI = 15) | Feta: Low (GI = 15) | Olive oil, garlic, parsley: Negligible GI

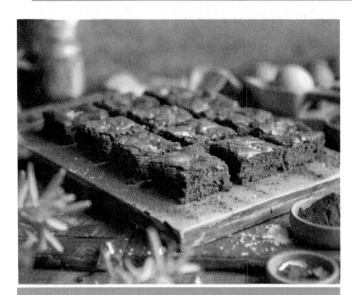

Coconut Flour Brownies

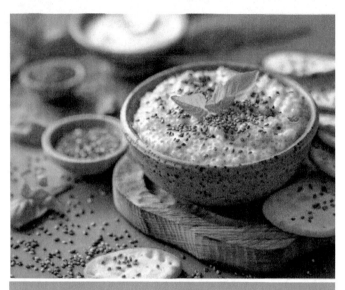

Vanilla Chia Seed Pudding

Prep: 15 mins | Cook: 20 mins | Serves: 8

Ingredients:

- 1/2 cup coconut flour (60g)
- 1/2 cup low carb sweeteners (100g)
- 1/4 cup cocoa powder (25g)
- 1/2 cup unsalted butter, melted (113g)
- 4 large eggs (200g)
- 1 tsp vanilla extract (5ml)
- 1/4 tsp salt (1g)

Instructions:

1. Preheat oven to 350°F (175°C).
2. In a bowl, mix coconut flour, low carb sweeteners, cocoa powder, and salt.
3. In another bowl, whisk melted butter, eggs, and vanilla extract.
4. Combine wet and dry ingredients, mixing until smooth.
5. Pour batter into a greased baking pan.
6. Bake for 20 minutes or until a toothpick inserted comes out clean. Cool before cutting into squares.

Nutritional Facts (Per Serving): Calories: 250 | Sugars: 2g | Fat: 11g | Carbohydrates: 28g | Protein: 12g | Fiber: 5g | Sodium: 100mg

Glycemic Index: Coconut flour: Low (GI = 45) | Low carb sweeteners: Negligible GI | Cocoa powder: Low (GI = 20) | Butter, eggs, vanilla extract, salt: Negligible GI

Prep: 5 mins | Cook: (Chill: 2 hours) | Serves: 2

Ingredients:

- 1 cup unsweetened almond milk (240ml)
- 1/4 cup chia seeds (40g)
- 1 tbsp low carb sweeteners (12g)
- 1 tsp vanilla extract (5ml)

Instructions:

1. In a bowl, combine almond milk, chia seeds, low carb sweeteners, and vanilla extract.
2. Stir well until the mixture is evenly combined.
3. Cover and refrigerate for at least 2 hours or overnight until it thickens. Serve chilled.

Nutritional Facts (Per Serving): Calories: 250 | Sugars: 2g | Fat: 11g | Carbohydrates: 29g | Protein: 12g | Fiber: 5g | Sodium: 150mg

Glycemic Index: Chia seeds: Low (GI = 1) | Almond milk: Low (GI = 15) | Vanilla extract: Negligible GI | Low carb sweeteners: Negligible GI

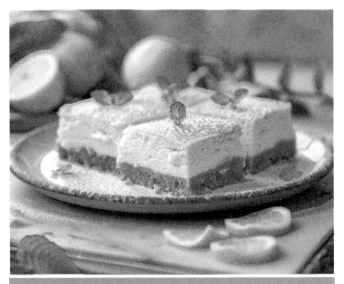

Low-Carb Lemon Cheesecake Bars

Prep: 20 mins | Cook: 25 mins | Serves: 8

Ingredients:

- 2 cups almond flour (240g)
- 1/2 cup low carb sweeteners (100g)
- 1/2 cup unsalted butter, melted (113g)
- 16 oz cream cheese, softened (450g)
- 3 large eggs (150g)
- 1/2 cup low carb sweeteners (100g)
- 1 tbsp lemon zest (6g)
- 1/4 cup lemon juice (60ml)
- 1 tsp vanilla extract (5ml)

Instructions:

1. Preheat oven to 350°F (175°C).
2. In a bowl, mix almond flour, 1/2 cup low carb sweeteners, and melted butter.
3. Press mixture into the bottom of a greased baking pan to form a crust.
4. Bake for 10 minutes and let cool.
5. In another bowl, beat cream cheese until smooth. Add eggs, 1/2 cup low carb sweeteners, lemon zest, lemon juice, and vanilla extract. Mix well.
6. Pour the cream cheese mixture over the cooled crust. Bake for 25 minutes or until set. Cool before cutting into bars.

Nutritional Facts (Per Serving): Calories: 250 | Sugars: 3g | Fat: 10g | Carbohydrates: 27g | Protein: 13g | Fiber: 4g | Sodium: 200mg

Glycemic Index: Almond flour: Low (GI = 1) | Low carb sweeteners: Negligible GI | Cream cheese: Low (GI = 15) | Lemon zest, lemon juice, vanilla extract, butter, eggs: Negligible GI

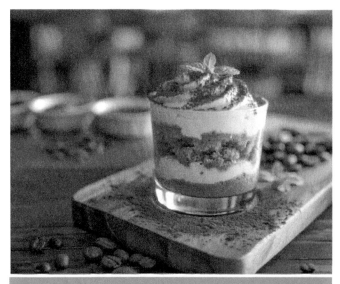

Low-Carb Tiramisu

Prep: 20 mins | Cook: 0 mins | Serves: 2

Ingredients:

- 1/2 cup mascarpone cheese (120g)
- 1/2 cup heavy cream (120ml)
- 1 tbsp low carb sweeteners (12g)
- 1 tsp vanilla extract (5ml)
- 1/2 cup brewed espresso, cooled (120ml)
- 2 tbsp cocoa powder (15g)
- 1/4 cup almond flour (30g)

Instructions:

1. In a bowl, beat mascarpone cheese, heavy cream, low carb sweeteners, and vanilla extract until smooth and fluffy.
2. In another bowl, mix brewed espresso and almond flour to create a sponge layer.
3. In serving glasses, layer the espresso-almond mixture and mascarpone cream mixture alternately, starting with the espresso-almond layer.
4. Dust the top layer with cocoa powder.
5. Chill for at least 1 hour before serving.

Nutritional Facts (Per Serving): Calories: 250 | Sugars: 3g | Fat: 10g | Carbohydrates: 28g | Protein: 13g | Fiber: 4g | Sodium: 200mg

Glycemic Index: Mascarpone cheese: Low (GI = 27) | Heavy cream: Low (GI = 1) | Cocoa powder: Low (GI = 20) | Almond flour: Low (GI = 1) | Espresso, vanilla extract, low carb sweeteners: Negligible GI

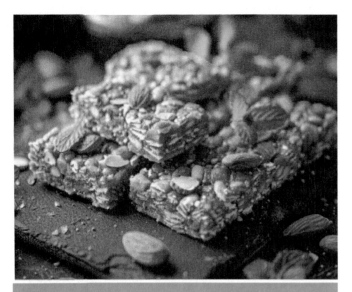

Vanilla Almond Protein Bars

Prep: 15 mins | Cook: 0 mins | Serves: 8

Ingredients:

- 1 cup almond flour (120g)
- 1/2 cup vanilla protein powder (60g)
- 1/4 cup almond butter (60g)
- 1/4 cup low carb sweeteners (50g)
- 1/4 cup unsweetened almond milk (60ml)
- 1 tsp vanilla extract (5ml)
- 1/4 cup sliced almonds (30g)

Instructions:

1. In a bowl, mix almond flour, vanilla protein powder, and low carb sweeteners.
2. Add almond butter, almond milk, and vanilla extract, stirring until well combined.
3. Press the mixture into a lined baking dish.
4. Sprinkle sliced almonds on top and press gently.
5. Refrigerate for at least 1 hour before cutting into bars.

Nutritional Facts (Per Serving): Calories: 250 | Sugars: 3g | Fat: 11g | Carbohydrates: 26g | Protein: 13g | Fiber: 5g | Sodium: 150mg

Glycemic Index: Almond flour: Low (GI = 1) | Vanilla protein powder: Low (GI = 15) | Almond butter: Low (GI = 1) | Almond milk: Low (GI = 15) | Low carb sweeteners: Negligible GI | Vanilla extract, sliced almonds: Negligible GI

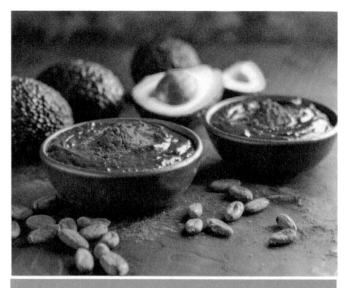

Chocolate Avocado Pudding

Prep: 10 mins | Cook: 0 mins | Serves: 2

Ingredients:

- 2 ripe avocados (400g)
- 1/4 cup unsweetened cocoa powder (25g)
- 1/4 cup low carb sweeteners (50g)
- 1/4 cup unsweetened almond milk (60ml)
- 1 tsp vanilla extract (5ml)

Instructions:

1. In a blender, combine avocados, cocoa powder, low carb sweeteners, almond milk, and vanilla extract.
2. Blend until smooth and creamy.
3. Divide the pudding into serving bowls and chill for at least 30 minutes before serving.

Nutritional Facts (Per Serving): Calories: 250 | Sugars: 3g | Fat: 11g | Carbohydrates: 28g | Protein: 12g | Fiber: 5g | Sodium: 200mg

Glycemic Index: Avocados: Low (GI = 10) | Cocoa powder: Low (GI = 20) | Almond milk: Low (GI = 15) | Vanilla extract, low carb sweeteners: Negligible GI

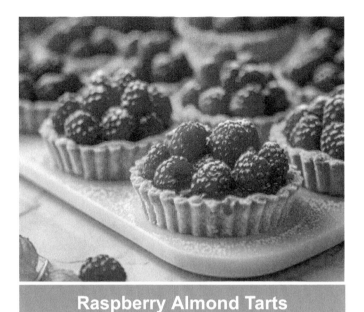

Raspberry Almond Tarts

Prep: 20 mins | Cook: 15 mins | Serves: 8

Ingredients:

- 1 cup almond flour (120g)
- 1/4 cup low carb sweeteners (50g)
- 1/4 cup unsalted butter, melted (60g)
- 1 large egg (50g)
- 1/2 tsp vanilla extract (2.5ml)
- 1 cup fresh raspberries (125g)

Instructions:

1. Preheat oven to 350°F (175°C).
2. In a bowl, mix almond flour, low carb sweeteners, melted butter, egg, and vanilla extract until well combined.
3. Press the mixture into tart molds or a muffin tin to form tart shells.
4. Bake for 10 minutes until lightly golden.
5. Fill each tart shell with fresh raspberries.
6. Bake for an additional 5 minutes.
7. Let cool before serving.

Nutritional Facts (Per Serving): Calories: 250 | Sugars: 3g | Fat: 11g | Carbohydrates: 29g | Protein: 12g | Fiber: 5g | Sodium: 100mg

Glycemic Index: Almond flour: Low (GI = 1) | Raspberries: Low (GI = 25) | Low carb sweeteners: Negligible GI | Butter, egg, vanilla extract: Negligible GI

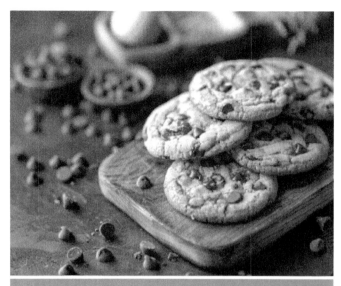

Low-Carb Chocolate Chip Cookies

Prep: 15 mins | Cook: 10 mins | Serves: 8

Ingredients:

- 1 cup almond flour (120g)
- 1/4 cup low carb sweeteners (50g)
- 1/4 cup unsalted butter, melted (60g)
- 1 large egg (50g)
- 1/2 tsp vanilla extract (2.5ml)
- 1/4 cup sugar-free chocolate chips (40g)

Instructions:

1. Preheat oven to 350°F (175°C).
2. In a bowl, mix almond flour, low carb sweeteners, melted butter, egg, and vanilla extract until well combined.
3. Fold in the sugar-free chocolate chips.
4. Drop spoonfuls of dough onto a baking sheet lined with parchment paper.
5. Flatten each cookie slightly.
6. Bake for 10 minutes until edges are golden.
7. Let cool before serving.

Nutritional Facts (Per Serving): Calories: 250 | Sugars: 3g | Fat: 10g | Carbohydrates: 28g | Protein: 12g | Fiber: 5g | Sodium: 150mg

Glycemic Index: Almond flour: Low (GI = 1) | Sugar-free chocolate chips: Low (GI = 1) | Low carb sweeteners: Negligible GI | Butter, egg, vanilla extract: Negligible GI

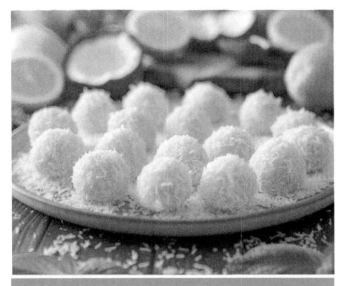

Lemon Coconut Balls

Prep: 15 mins | Cook: 0 mins | Serves: 8

Ingredients:

- 1 cup shredded unsweetened coconut (80g)
- 1/2 cup almond flour (60g)
- 1/4 cup low carb sweeteners (50g)
- 1/4 cup coconut oil, melted (60ml)
- 1 tbsp lemon zest (6g)
- 2 tbsp lemon juice (30ml)
- 1 tsp vanilla extract (5ml)

Instructions:

1. In a bowl, mix shredded coconut, almond flour, and low carb sweeteners.
2. Add melted coconut oil, lemon zest, lemon juice, and vanilla extract. Mix until well combined.
3. Roll the mixture into small balls and place them on a baking sheet lined with parchment paper.
4. Refrigerate for at least 1 hour before serving.

Nutritional Facts (Per Serving): Calories: 250 | Sugars: 2g | Fat: 11g | Carbohydrates: 28g | Protein: 12g | Fiber: 5g | Sodium: 100mg

Glycemic Index: Coconut: Low (GI = 45) | Almond flour: Low (GI = 1) | Low carb sweeteners: Negligible GI | Coconut oil, lemon zest, lemon juice, vanilla extract: Negligible GI

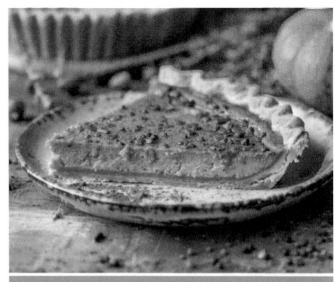

Low-Carb Pumpkin Pie

Prep: 15 mins | Cook: 40 mins | Serves: 8

Ingredients:

- 1 cup almond flour (120g)
- 1/4 cup coconut flour (30g)
- 1/4 cup low carb sweeteners (50g)
- 1/4 cup unsalted butter, melted (60g)
- 1 cup pumpkin puree (240g)
- 1/2 cup heavy cream (120ml)
- 2 large eggs (100g)
- 1/4 cup low carb sweeteners (50g)
- 1 tsp vanilla extract (5ml)
- 1 tsp ground cinnamon (2g)
- 1/2 tsp ground nutmeg (1g)
- 1/4 tsp ground ginger (0.5g)
- 1/4 tsp salt (1g)

Instructions:

1. Preheat oven to 350°F (175°C).
2. In a bowl, mix almond flour, coconut flour, and low carb sweeteners with melted butter. Press into a pie dish to form the crust.
3. In another bowl, mix pumpkin puree, heavy cream, eggs, low carb sweeteners, vanilla extract, cinnamon, nutmeg, ginger, and salt.
4. Pour the pumpkin mixture into the crust.
5. Bake for 40 minutes or until the filling is set.
6. Let cool before serving.

Nutritional Facts (Per Serving): Calories: 250 | Sugars: 3g | Fat: 10g | Carbohydrates: 29g | Protein: 13g | Fiber: 5g | Sodium: 150mg

Glycemic Index: Pumpkin: Low (GI = 75) | Almond flour: Low (GI = 1) | Coconut flour: Low (GI = 51) | Low carb sweeteners: Negligible GI | Heavy cream, eggs, vanilla extract, spices, salt: Negligible GI

CHAPTER 15: DESSERTS: Low-carb Baking Ideas

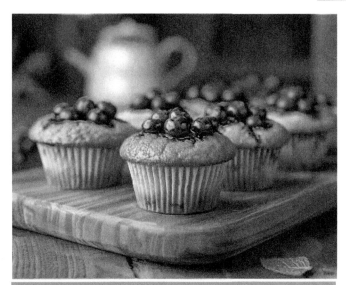

Almond Flour Blueberry Muffins

Prep: 15 mins | Cook: 20 mins | Serves: 8

Ingredients:

- 2 cups almond flour (240g)
- 1/4 cup low carb sweeteners (50g)
- 1/2 tsp baking powder (2g)
- 1/4 tsp salt (1g)
- 3 large eggs (150g)
- 1/4 cup unsweetened almond milk (60ml)
- 1 tsp vanilla extract (5ml)
- 1 cup fresh blueberries (150g)

Instructions:

1. Preheat oven to 350°F (175°C).
2. In a bowl, mix almond flour, low carb sweeteners, baking powder, and salt.
3. In another bowl, whisk eggs, almond milk, and vanilla extract. Combine wet and dry ingredients, then fold in blueberries. Divide the batter evenly into a lined muffin tin.
4. Bake for 20 minutes or until a toothpick inserted comes out clean. Let cool before serving.

Nutritional Facts (Per Serving): Calories: 250 | Sugars: 3g | Fat: 11g | Carbohydrates: 29g | Protein: 13g | Fiber: 5g | Sodium: 150mg

Glycemic Index: Almond flour: Low (GI = 1) | Blueberries: Low (GI = 25) | Low carb sweeteners: Negligible GI | Almond milk, eggs, vanilla extract: Negligible GI

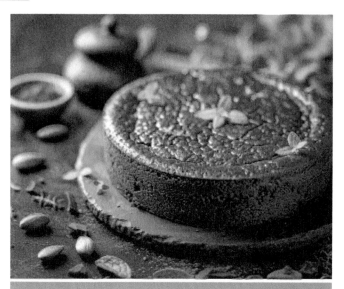

Coconut Flour Chocolate Cake

Prep: 15 mins | Cook: 25 mins | Serves: 8

Ingredients:

- 1/2 cup coconut flour (60g)
- 1/4 cup unsweetened cocoa powder (25g)
- 1/2 cup low carb sweeteners (100g)
- 1/2 tsp baking powder (2g)
- 1/4 tsp salt (1g)
- 4 large eggs (200g)
- 1/2 cup unsweetened almond milk (120ml)
- 1/4 cup melted coconut oil (60ml)
- 1 tsp vanilla extract (5ml)

Instructions:

1. Preheat oven to 350°F (175°C).
2. In a bowl, mix coconut flour, cocoa powder, low carb sweeteners, baking powder, and salt.
3. In another bowl, whisk eggs, almond milk, melted coconut oil, and vanilla extract.
4. Combine wet and dry ingredients until smooth.
5. Pour the batter into a greased cake pan.
6. Bake for 25 minutes or until a toothpick inserted comes out clean. Let cool before serving.

Nutritional Facts (Per Serving): Calories: 250 | Sugars: 3g | Fat: 10g | Carbohydrates: 29g | Protein: 12g | Fiber: 5g | Sodium: 150mg

Glycemic Index: Coconut flour: Low (GI = 51) | Cocoa powder: Low (GI = 20) | Low carb sweeteners: Negligible GI | Almond milk, eggs, coconut oil, vanilla extract: Negligible GI

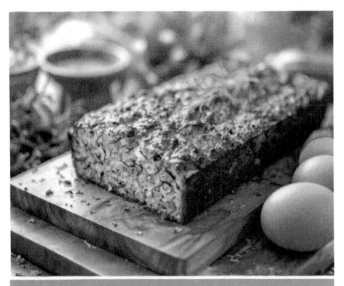

Keto Zucchini Bread

Prep: 15 mins | Cook: 45 mins | Serves: 8

Ingredients:

- 1 1/2 cups almond flour (180g)
- 1/4 cup coconut flour (30g)
- 1/2 cup low carb sweeteners (100g)
- 1 tsp baking powder (5g)
- 1/2 tsp salt (2.5g)
- 1 tsp cinnamon (2g)
- 3 large eggs (150g)
- 1/4 cup melted coconut oil (60ml)
- 1 tsp vanilla extract (5ml)
- 1 cup grated zucchini (150g)

Instructions:

1. Preheat oven to 350°F (175°C).
2. In a bowl, mix almond flour, coconut flour, low carb sweeteners, baking powder, salt, and cinnamon.
3. In another bowl, whisk eggs, coconut oil, and vanilla extract.
4. Combine wet and dry ingredients, then fold in grated zucchini.
5. Pour batter into a greased loaf pan.
6. Bake for 45 minutes or until a toothpick inserted comes out clean.
7. Let cool before slicing.

Nutritional Facts (Per Serving): Calories: 250 | Sugars: 3g | Fat: 10g | Carbohydrates: 29g | Protein: 12g | Fiber: 5g | Sodium: 150mg

Glycemic Index: Almond flour: Low (GI = 1) | Zucchini: Low (GI = 15) | Coconut flour: Low (GI = 51) | Low carb sweeteners: Negligible GI | Coconut oil, eggs, vanilla extract: Negligible GI

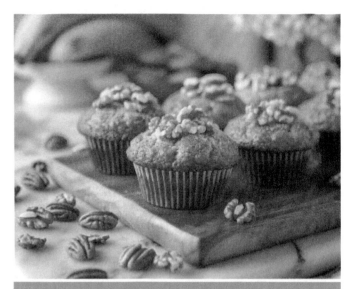

Low-Carb Banana Nut Muffins

Prep: 15 mins | Cook: 20 mins | Serves: 8

Ingredients:

- 1 1/2 cups almond flour (180g)
- 1/4 cup coconut flour (30g)
- 1/2 cup low carb sweeteners (100g)
- 1 tsp baking powder (5g)
- 1/2 tsp salt (2.5g)
- 3 large eggs (150g)
- 1/4 cup melted butter (60g)
- 1 tsp vanilla extract (5ml)
- 1/2 cup mashed banana (120g)
- 1/4 cup chopped walnuts (30g)

Instructions:

1. Preheat oven to 350°F (175°C).
2. In a bowl, mix almond flour, coconut flour, low carb sweeteners, baking powder, and salt.
3. In another bowl, whisk eggs, melted butter, and vanilla extract.
4. Combine wet and dry ingredients, then fold in mashed banana and chopped walnuts.
5. Divide the batter into a lined muffin tin.
6. Bake for 20 minutes or until a toothpick inserted comes out clean.
7. Let cool before serving.

Nutritional Facts (Per Serving): Calories: 250 | Sugars: 3g | Fat: 11g | Carbohydrates: 29g | Protein: 13g | Fiber: 5g | Sodium: 150mg

Glycemic Index: Almond flour: Low (GI = 1) | Banana: Low (GI = 51) | Coconut flour: Low (GI = 51) | Low carb sweeteners: Negligible GI | Butter, eggs, vanilla extract, walnuts: Negligible GI

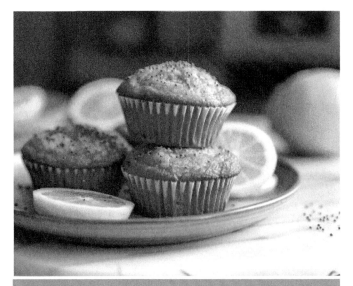

Sugar-Free Lemon Poppy Seed Muffins

Prep: 15 mins | Cook: 20 mins | Serves: 8

Ingredients:

- 1 1/2 cups almond flour (180g)
- 1/4 cup coconut flour (30g)
- 1/2 cup low carb sweeteners (100g)
- 1 tsp baking powder (5g)
- 1/4 tsp salt (1g)
- 3 large eggs (150g)
- 1/4 cup unsweetened almond milk (60ml)
- 1/4 cup melted coconut oil (60ml)
- 1 tbsp poppy seeds (10g)
- 1 tbsp lemon zest (6g)
- 1/4 cup lemon juice (60ml)

Instructions:

1. Preheat oven to 350°F (175°C).
2. In a bowl, mix almond flour, coconut flour, low carb sweeteners, baking powder, salt, and poppy seeds.
3. In another bowl, whisk eggs, almond milk, melted coconut oil, lemon zest, and lemon juice.
4. Combine wet and dry ingredients.
5. Divide the batter evenly into a lined muffin tin.
6. Bake for 20 minutes or until a toothpick inserted comes out clean. Let cool before serving.

Nutritional Facts (Per Serving): Calories: 250 | Sugars: 3g | Fat: 10g | Carbohydrates: 29g | Protein: 13g | Fiber: 5g | Sodium: 150mg

Glycemic Index: Almond flour: Low (GI = 1) | Poppy seeds: Low (GI = 15) | Coconut flour: Low (GI = 51) | Low carb sweeteners: Negligible GI | Almond milk, eggs, coconut oil, lemon zest, lemon juice: Negligible GI

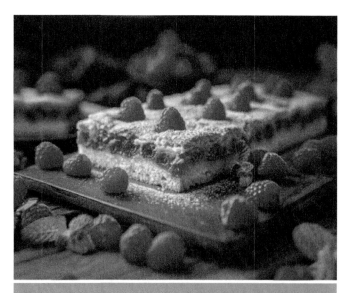

Almond Flour Raspberry Bars

Prep: 15 mins | Cook: 30 mins | Serves: 8

Ingredients:

- 2 cups almond flour (240g)
- 1/2 cup low carb sweeteners (100g)
- 1/4 cup unsalted butter, melted (60g)
- 1/4 tsp salt (1g)
- 1 tsp vanilla extract (5ml)
- 1 cup fresh raspberries (150g)

Instructions:

1. Preheat oven to 350°F (175°C).
2. In a bowl, mix almond flour, low carb sweeteners, melted butter, salt, and vanilla extract.
3. Press half of the mixture into the bottom of a greased baking pan to form the crust.
4. Spread raspberries evenly over the crust.
5. Sprinkle the remaining almond flour mixture on top of the raspberries.
6. Bake for 30 minutes or until the top is golden.
7. Let cool before cutting into bars.

Nutritional Facts (Per Serving): Calories: 250 | Sugars: 3g | Fat: 11g | Carbohydrates: 29g | Protein: 12g | Fiber: 5g | Sodium: 150mg

Glycemic Index: Almond flour: Low (GI = 1) | Raspberries: Low (GI = 25) | Low carb sweeteners: Negligible GI | Butter, vanilla extract: Negligible GI

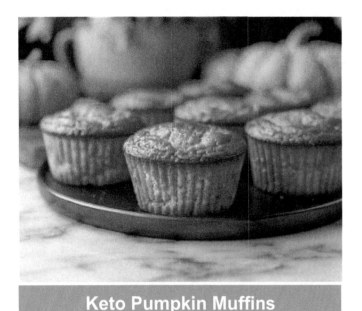

Keto Pumpkin Muffins

Prep: 15 mins | Cook: 20 mins | Serves: 8

Ingredients:

- 1 1/2 cups almond flour (180g)
- 1/4 cup coconut flour (30g)
- 1/2 cup pumpkin puree (120g)
- 1/2 cup low carb sweeteners (100g)
- 3 large eggs (150g)
- 1/4 cup melted coconut oil (60ml)
- 1 tsp vanilla extract (5ml)
- 1 tsp baking powder (5g)
- 1/2 tsp cinnamon (2g)
- 1/4 tsp nutmeg (1g)
- 1/4 tsp salt (1g)

Instructions:

1. Preheat oven to 350°F (175°C).
2. In a bowl, mix almond flour, coconut flour, low carb sweeteners, baking powder, cinnamon, nutmeg, and salt.
3. In another bowl, whisk pumpkin puree, eggs, melted coconut oil, and vanilla extract.
4. Combine wet and dry ingredients.
5. Divide the batter evenly into a lined muffin tin.
6. Bake for 20 minutes or until a toothpick inserted comes out clean.

Nutritional Facts (Per Serving): Calories: 250 | Sugars: 3g | Fat: 10g | Carbohydrates: 29g | Protein: 13g | Fiber: 5g | Sodium: 150mg

Glycemic Index: Almond flour: Low (GI = 1) | Pumpkin: Low (GI = 75) | Coconut flour: Low (GI = 51) | Low carb sweeteners: Negligible GI | Coconut oil, eggs, vanilla extract, spices: Negligible GI

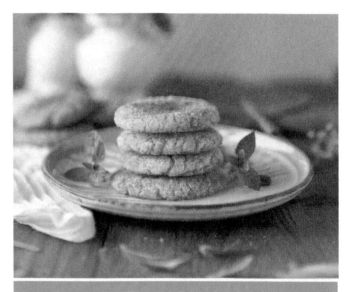

Almond Flour Snickerdoodle Cookies

Prep: 15 mins | Cook: 10 mins | Serves: 8

Ingredients:

- 1 1/2 cups almond flour (180g)
- 1/4 cup low carb sweeteners (50g)
- 1/4 cup melted butter (60g)
- 1 large egg (50g)
- 1 tsp vanilla extract (5ml)
- 1/2 tsp baking powder (2g)
- 1/4 tsp salt (1g)
- 1 tsp cinnamon (2g)

Instructions:

1. Preheat oven to 350°F (175°C).
2. In a bowl, mix almond flour, low carb sweeteners, baking powder, salt, and cinnamon.
3. In another bowl, whisk melted butter, egg, and vanilla extract. Combine wet and dry ingredients until a dough forms.
4. Roll dough into small balls and place on a baking sheet lined with parchment paper. Flatten each ball slightly.
5. Bake for 10 minutes or until edges are golden.

Nutritional Facts (Per Serving): Calories: 250 | Sugars: 3g | Fat: 11g | Carbohydrates: 29g | Protein: 12g | Fiber: 5g | Sodium: 150mg

Glycemic Index: Almond flour: Low (GI = 1) | Low carb sweeteners: Negligible GI | Butter, eggs, vanilla extract, cinnamon: Negligible GI

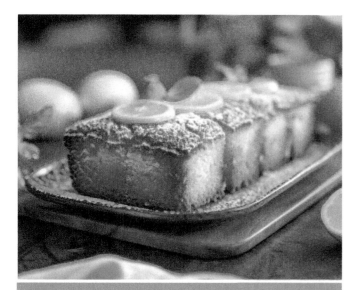

Lemon Pound Cake with Almond Flour

Prep: 15 mins | Cook: 40 mins | Serves: 8

Ingredients:

- 2 cups almond flour (240g)
- 1/2 cup low carb sweeteners (100g)
-
- 4 large eggs (200g)
- 1/4 cup unsweetened almond milk (60ml)
- 2 tbsp lemon zest (12g)
- 1/4 cup lemon juice (60ml)
- 1 tsp vanilla extract (5ml)
- 1 tsp baking powder (5g)
- 1/4 tsp salt (1g)
- 1/4 cup coconut flour (30g)
- 1/4 cup melted butter (60g)

Instructions:

1. Preheat oven to 350°F (175°C).
2. In a bowl, mix almond flour, coconut flour, low carb sweeteners, baking powder, and salt.
3. In another bowl, whisk melted butter, eggs, almond milk, lemon zest, lemon juice, and vanilla extract.
4. Combine wet and dry ingredients.
5. Pour batter into a greased loaf pan.
6. Bake for 40 minutes or until a toothpick inserted comes out clean. Let cool before serving.

Nutritional Facts (Per Serving): Calories: 250 | Sugars: 3g | Fat: 11g | Carbohydrates: 29g | Protein: 13g | Fiber: 5g | Sodium: 150mg

Glycemic Index: Almond flour: Low (GI = 1) | Coconut flour: Low (GI = 51) | Low carb sweeteners: Negligible GI | Butter, eggs, almond milk, lemon zest, lemon juice, vanilla extract: Negligible GI

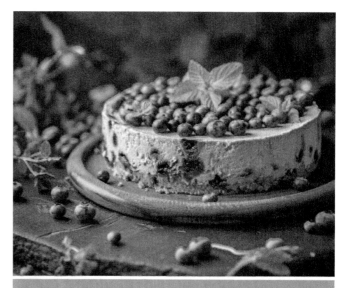

Keto Blueberry Cheesecake

Prep: 20 mins | Cook: 60 mins | Serves: 8

Ingredients:

- 2 cups almond flour (240g)
- 1/4 cup melted butter (60g)
- 1/2 cup low carb sweeteners (100g) (divided)
- 16 oz cream cheese, softened (450g)
- 3 large eggs (150g)
- 1/2 cup sour cream (120g)
- 1 tsp vanilla extract (5ml)
- 1 cup fresh blueberries (150g)

Instructions:

1. Preheat oven to 325°F (160°C).
2. In a bowl, mix almond flour, 1/4 cup low carb sweeteners, and melted butter. Press mixture into the bottom of a springform pan to form a crust.
3. In another bowl, beat cream cheese and remaining 1/4 cup low carb sweeteners until smooth. Add eggs one at a time, beating after each addition.
4. Mix in sour cream and vanilla extract until well combined. Pour cheesecake batter over the crust. Sprinkle blueberries on top. Bake for 60 minutes or until set. Let cool before serving.

Nutritional Facts (Per Serving): Calories: 250 | Sugars: 4g | Fat: 10g | Carbohydrates: 29g | Protein: 13g | Fiber: 5g | Sodium: 200mg

Glycemic Index: Almond flour: Low (GI = 1) | Blueberries: Low (GI = 25) | Low carb sweeteners: Negligible GI | Cream cheese, butter, eggs, sour cream, vanilla extract: Negligible GI

CHAPTER 16: DINNERS: Healthy Sides And Vegetables

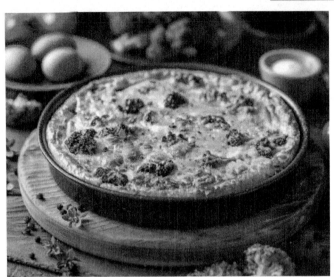

Broccoli and Cheddar Cheese Egg Bake

Prep: 15 mins | Cook: 30 mins | Serves: 4

Ingredients:

- 4 cups broccoli florets (450g)
- 1 cup shredded cheddar cheese (120g)
- 8 large eggs (400g)
- 1/2 cup milk (120ml)
- 1 tsp low carb sweeteners
- 1 tsp salt (5g)
- 1/2 tsp black pepper (2.5g)

Instructions:

1. Preheat the oven to 375°F (190°C).
2. Steam the broccoli florets until tender, about 5 minutes. In a large bowl, whisk together the eggs, milk, low carb sweeteners, salt, and pepper.
3. Mix in the steamed broccoli and shredded cheddar cheese.
4. Pour the mixture into a greased baking dish.
5. Bake in the preheated oven for 25-30 minutes, or until the center is set and the top is golden brown.
6. Let cool slightly before serving.

Nutritional Facts (Per Serving): Calories: 350 | Sugars: 5g | Fat: 14g | Carbohydrates: 10g | Protein: 20g | Fiber: 6g | Sodium: 480mg

Glycemic Index: Broccoli: Low (GI = 10) | Cheddar Cheese: Negligible GI (no carbs) | Eggs: Negligible GI (no carbs) | Milk: Low (GI = 30)

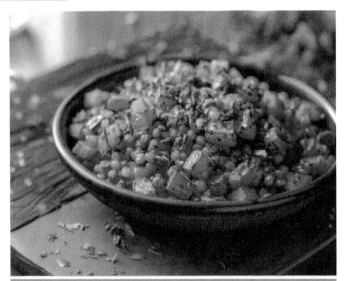

Barley and Roasted Root Vegetable Salad

Prep: 20 mins | Cook: 40 mins | Serves: 4

Ingredients:

- 1 cup pearl barley (200g)
- 2 cups diced carrots (250g)
- 2 cups diced parsnips (250g)
- 1 cup diced red onion (150g)
- 2 tbsp olive oil (30ml)
- 1 tsp low carb sweeteners
- 1 tsp salt (5g)
- 1/2 tsp black pepper (2.5g)
- 1 tbsp chopped fresh parsley (15g)

Instructions:

1. Preheat oven to 400°F (200°C).
2. Cook barley according to package instructions.
3. Toss carrots, parsnips, and red onion with olive oil, sweetener, salt, and pepper.
4. Roast vegetables on a baking sheet for 30-35 minutes until tender and golden brown.
5. Combine cooked barley and roasted vegetables in a large bowl.
6. Sprinkle with chopped fresh parsley and mix well.

Nutritional Facts (Per Serving): Calories: 350 | Sugars: 6g | Fat: 13g | Carbohydrates: 45g | Protein: 19g | Fiber: 7g | Sodium: 470mg

Glycemic Index: Pearl Barley: Medium (GI = 25) | Carrots: Medium (GI = 35) | Parsnips: Medium (GI = 52) | Red Onion: Low (GI = 10)

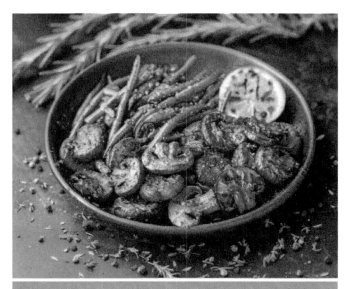

Grilled Green Beans with Lemon Zest and Mushrooms

Prep: 10 mins | Cook: 15 mins | Serves: 4

Ingredients:

- 1.5 lbs green beans (675g)
- 12 oz mushrooms, sliced (340g)
- 1/4 cup olive oil (60ml)
- Zest of 2 lemons
- 1.5 tsp salt (7.5g)
- 1 tsp black pepper (5g)
- 2 oz grated Parmesan cheese (60g)

Instructions:

1. Preheat the grill to medium-high heat.
2. Toss green beans and mushrooms with olive oil, lemon zest, salt, and pepper.
3. Place green beans and mushrooms on the grill. Cook for 10-15 minutes, turning occasionally, until tender and slightly charred.
4. Remove from the grill and place in a serving dish.
5. Sprinkle with grated Parmesan cheese before serving.

Nutritional Facts (Per Serving): Calories: 350 | Sugars: 7g | Fat: 14g | Carbohydrates: 38g | Protein: 20g | Fiber: 7g | Sodium: 450mg

Glycemic Index: Green Beans: Low (GI = 15) | Mushrooms: Low (GI = 15) | Lemon Zest: Negligible GI | Parmesan Cheese: Low (GI = 27)

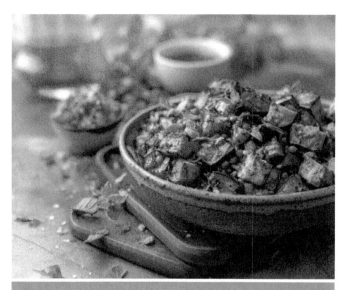

Eggplant and Lentil Salad with Mint Yogurt Dressing

Prep: 20 mins | Cook: 25 mins | Serves: 4

Ingredients:

- 1 large eggplant, diced (450g)
- 1 cup cooked lentils (200g)
- 1/2 cup diced red onion (75g)
- 1/4 cup chopped fresh mint (15g)
- 1 cup Greek yogurt (240g)
- 1 tbsp lemon juice (15ml)
- 1 tsp low carb sweeteners
- 1 tsp salt (5g)
- 1/2 tsp black pepper (2.5g)
- 2 tbsp olive oil (30ml)

Instructions:

1. Preheat the oven to 400°F (200°C).
2. Toss diced eggplant with olive oil, salt, and pepper.
3. Spread eggplant on a baking sheet and roast for 20-25 minutes, until tender and slightly browned.
4. In a large bowl, combine roasted eggplant, cooked lentils, and red onion.
5. In a small bowl, mix Greek yogurt, lemon juice, low carb sweeteners, chopped mint, salt, and pepper to make the dressing.
6. Pour the mint yogurt dressing over the eggplant and lentil mixture, and toss to combine.

Nutritional Facts (Per Serving): Calories: 350 | Sugars: 6g | Fat: 13g | Carbohydrates: 45g | Protein: 19g | Fiber: 7g | Sodium: 480mg

Glycemic Index: Eggplant: Low (GI = 15) | Lentils: Low (GI = 32) | Greek Yogurt: Low (GI = 35) | Mint: Negligible GI

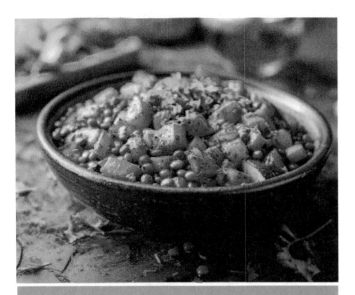

Warm Lentil and Roasted Veggie Salad

Prep: 20 mins | Cook: 30 mins | Serves: 4

Ingredients:

- 1 cup dried green lentils (200g)
- 2 cups diced carrots (250g)
- 2 cups diced zucchini (250g)
- 1 red bell pepper, diced (150g)
- 2 tbsp olive oil (30ml)
- 1 tsp salt (5g)
- 1/2 tsp black pepper (2.5g)
- 1/4 cup chopped fresh parsley (15g)
- 2 tbsp balsamic vinegar (30ml)
- 1 tsp low carb sweeteners

Instructions:

1. Preheat the oven to 400°F (200°C).
2. Cook the lentils according to package instructions, then drain and set aside.
3. Toss the carrots, zucchini, and red bell pepper with 1 tbsp olive oil, 1/2 tsp salt, and 1/4 tsp black pepper. Spread on a baking sheet and roast for 25-30 minutes until tender and slightly caramelized.
4. In a large bowl, combine cooked lentils, roasted vegetables, chopped parsley, balsamic vinegar, remaining olive oil, low carb sweeteners, remaining salt, and pepper. Toss well.

Nutritional Facts (Per Serving): Calories: 350 | Sugars: 6g | Fat: 14g | Carbohydrates: 45g | Protein: 19g | Fiber: 7g | Sodium: 480mg

Glycemic Index: Lentils: Low (GI = 32) | Carrots: Medium (GI = 35) | Zucchini: Low (GI = 15) | Red Bell Pepper: Low (GI = 15)

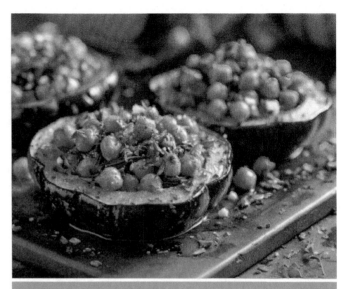

Chickpea and Spinach Stuffed Acorn Squash

Prep: 20 mins | Cook: 40 mins | Serves: 4

Ingredients:

- 2 medium acorn squashes, halved and seeded (800g)
- 1 cup cooked chickpeas (200g)
- 4 cups fresh spinach (120g)
- 1/2 cup diced red onion (75g)
- 2 tbsp olive oil (30ml)
- 1 tsp ground cumin (5g)
- 1 tsp salt (5g)
- 1/2 tsp black pepper (2.5g)
- 1/4 cup crumbled feta cheese (60g)
- 1 tbsp lemon juice (15ml)

Instructions:

1. Preheat oven to 400°F (200°C). Brush acorn squash halves with 1 tbsp olive oil, season with half the salt and pepper. Roast cut side down on a baking sheet for 30-40 minutes until tender.
2. Sauté diced red onion in remaining olive oil over medium heat until softened.
3. Add chickpeas, spinach, cumin, remaining salt, and pepper; cook until spinach wilts and chickpeas are heated through. Stir in lemon juice.
4. Fill each roasted squash half with the chickpea and spinach mixture.
5. Top with crumbled feta cheese and serve.

Nutritional Facts (Per Serving): Calories: 350 | Sugars: 7g | Fat: 14g | Carbohydrates: 45g | Protein: 18g | Fiber: 7g | Sodium: 490mg

Glycemic Index: Acorn Squash: Medium (GI = 50) | Chickpeas: Low (GI = 28) | Spinach: Low (GI = 15) | Feta Cheese: Low (GI = 15)

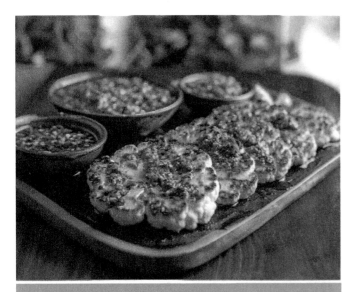

Roasted Cauliflower Steaks with Chimichurri Sauce

Prep: 15 mins | Cook: 30 mins | Serves: 4

Ingredients:

- 2 large cauliflower heads (1200g)
- 4 tbsp olive oil (60ml)
- 1 tsp salt (5g)
- 1/2 tsp black pepper (2.5g)
- 1 cup fresh parsley, chopped (60g)
- 1/4 cup fresh cilantro, chopped (15g)
- 4 cloves garlic, minced (12g)
- 1/4 cup red wine vinegar (60ml)
- 1/2 tsp red pepper flakes (2.5g)

Instructions:

1. Preheat the oven to 425°F (220°C).
2. Slice cauliflower heads into 1-inch thick steaks. Brush both sides with 2 tbsp olive oil, and season with 1/2 tsp salt and 1/4 tsp black pepper.
3. Place cauliflower steaks on a baking sheet and roast for 25-30 minutes, flipping halfway through, until golden and tender.
4. In a bowl, combine parsley, cilantro, garlic, red wine vinegar, remaining olive oil, red pepper flakes, and remaining salt and pepper to make the chimichurri sauce.
5. Drizzle chimichurri sauce over roasted cauliflower steaks before serving.

Nutritional Facts (Per Serving): Calories: 350 | Sugars: 6g | Fat: 14g | Carbohydrates: 45g | Protein: 20g | Fiber: 7g | Sodium: 480mg

Glycemic Index: Cauliflower: Low (GI = 15) | Olive Oil: Negligible GI | Parsley: Low (GI = 5) | Cilantro: Low (GI = 5)

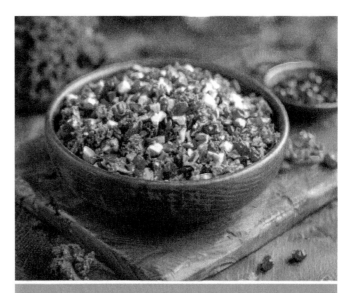

Wild Rice and Kale Salad with Cranberries

Prep: 20 mins | Cook: 45 mins | Serves: 4

Ingredients:

- 1 cup wild rice (200g)
- 4 cups chopped kale (120g)
- 1/2 cup dried cranberries (60g)
- 1/4 cup chopped walnuts (30g)
- 1/4 cup feta cheese, crumbled (60g)
- 2 tbsp olive oil (30ml)
- 2 tbsp apple cider vinegar (30ml)
- 1 tsp low carb sweeteners
- 1 tsp salt (5g)
- 1/2 tsp black pepper (2.5g)

Instructions:

1. Cook wild rice according to package instructions, then set aside to cool.
2. In a large bowl, combine chopped kale, dried cranberries, chopped walnuts, and crumbled feta cheese.
3. In a small bowl, whisk together olive oil, apple cider vinegar, low carb sweeteners, salt, and black pepper.
4. Pour the dressing over the kale mixture and toss to combine.
5. Add cooled wild rice to the salad and mix well.
6. Serve chilled or at room temperature.

Nutritional Facts (Per Serving): Calories: 350 | Sugars: 7g | Fat: 15g | Carbohydrates: 45g | Protein: 18g | Fiber: 7g | Sodium: 480mg

Glycemic Index: Wild Rice: Medium (GI = 45) | Kale: Low (GI = 2-4) | Cranberries: Low (GI = 45) | Walnuts: Low (GI = 15) | Feta Cheese: Low (GI = 15)

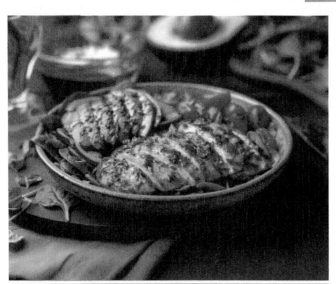

Spinach and Grilled Chicken Salad with Avocado

Prep: 15 mins | Cook: 0 mins | Serves: 4

Ingredients:

- 4 cups fresh spinach (120g)
- 2 grilled chicken breasts, sliced (300g)
- 1 avocado, diced (150g)
- 1/2 cup cherry tomatoes, halved (75g)
- 1/4 cup red onion, thinly sliced (35g)
- 2 tbsp olive oil (30ml)
- 1 tbsp lemon juice (15ml)
- 1 tsp Dijon mustard (5g)
- 1 tsp low carb sweeteners
- 1 tsp salt (5g)
- 1/2 tsp black pepper (2.5g)

Instructions:

1. In a large bowl, combine fresh spinach, sliced grilled chicken breasts, diced avocado, cherry tomatoes, and thinly sliced red onion.
2. In a small bowl, whisk together olive oil, lemon juice, Dijon mustard, low carb sweeteners, salt, and black pepper to make the dressing.
3. Pour the dressing over the salad and toss to combine.

Nutritional Facts (Per Serving): Calories: 350 | Sugars: 5g | Fat: 15g | Carbohydrates: 35g | Protein: 22g | Fiber: 7g | Sodium: 470mg

Glycemic Index: Spinach: Low (GI = 2-5) | Chicken: Negligible GI | Avocado: Low (GI = 15) | Cherry Tomatoes: Low (GI = 15)

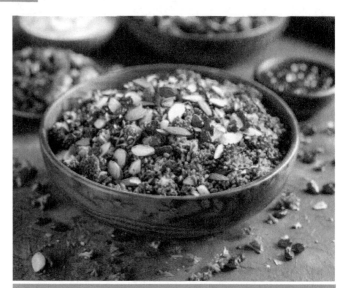

Broccoli and Cranberry Salad with Almonds

Prep: 15 mins | Cook: 0 mins | Serves: 4

Ingredients:

- 4 cups chopped broccoli (600g)
- 1/2 cup dried cranberries (60g)
- 1/4 cup sliced almonds (30g)
- 1/2 cup Greek yogurt (120g)
- 2 tbsp apple cider vinegar (30ml)
- 1 tbsp low carb sweeteners
- 1 tsp salt (5g)
- 1/2 tsp black pepper (2.5g)

Instructions:

1. In a large bowl, combine chopped broccoli, dried cranberries, and sliced almonds.
2. In a small bowl, whisk together Greek yogurt, apple cider vinegar, low carb sweeteners, salt, and black pepper to make the dressing.
3. Pour the dressing over the broccoli mixture and toss to combine.
4. Serve immediately or chill before serving.

Nutritional Facts (Per Serving): Calories: 350 | Sugars: 7g | Fat: 14g | Carbohydrates: 40g | Protein: 20g | Fiber: 7g | Sodium: 480mg

Glycemic Index: Broccoli: Low (GI = 10) | Cranberries: Low (GI = 45) | Almonds: Low (GI = 15) | Greek Yogurt: Low (GI = 35)

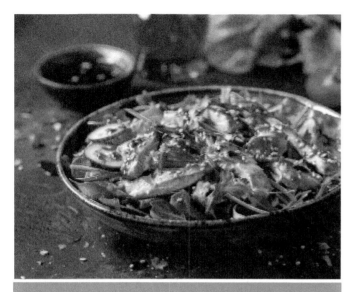

Asian-Inspired Chicken Salad with Sesame Dressing

Prep: 20 mins | Cook: 0 mins | Serves: 4

Ingredients:

- 2 cups shredded cooked chicken (250g)
- 4 cups mixed salad greens (120g)
- 1 cup shredded carrots (100g)
- 1 cup sliced cucumbers (120g)
- 1 red bell pepper, thinly sliced (150g)
- 1/4 cup chopped cilantro (15g)
- 2 tbsp sesame seeds (30g)
- 3 tbsp soy sauce (45ml)
- 2 tbsp rice vinegar (30ml)
- 1 tbsp sesame oil (15ml)
- 1 tbsp low carb sweeteners
- 1 clove garlic, minced (3g)
- 1 tsp grated ginger (5g)

Instructions:

1. In a large bowl, combine shredded chicken, salad greens, shredded carrots, sliced cucumbers, red bell pepper, and chopped cilantro.
2. In a small bowl, whisk together soy sauce, rice vinegar, sesame oil, low carb sweeteners, minced garlic, and grated ginger to make the dressing.
3. Pour the sesame dressing over the salad and toss to combine.
4. Sprinkle with sesame seeds before serving.

Nutritional Facts (Per Serving): Calories: 350 | Sugars: 5g | Fat: 14g | Carbohydrates: 40g | Protein: 20g | Fiber: 7g | Sodium: 480mg

Glycemic Index: Chicken: Negligible GI | Salad Greens: Low (GI = 2-5) | Carrots: Medium (GI = 35) | Cucumbers: Low (GI = 15) | Red Bell Pepper: Low (GI = 15)

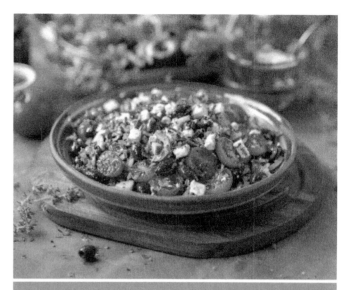

Greek Salad with Kalamata Olives and Feta

Prep: 15 mins | Cook: 0 mins | Serves: 4

Ingredients:

- 4 cups chopped romaine lettuce (200g)
- 1 cup cherry tomatoes, halved (150g)
- 1 cucumber, diced (200g)
- 1/2 red onion, thinly sliced (75g)
- 1/2 cup Kalamata olives (70g)
- 1/2 cup crumbled feta cheese (60g)
- 1/4 cup extra virgin olive oil (60ml)
- 2 tbsp red wine vinegar (30ml)
- 1 tsp dried oregano (5g)
- 1 tsp salt (5g)
- 1/2 tsp black pepper (2.5g)

Instructions:

1. In a large bowl, combine chopped romaine lettuce, cherry tomatoes, diced cucumber, thinly sliced red onion, Kalamata olives, and crumbled feta cheese.
2. In a small bowl, whisk together extra virgin olive oil, red wine vinegar, dried oregano, salt, and black pepper to make the dressing.
3. Pour the dressing over the salad and toss to combine.

Nutritional Facts (Per Serving): Calories: 350 | Sugars: 6g | Fat: 15g | Carbohydrates: 35g | Protein: 18g | Fiber: 7g | Sodium: 480mg

Glycemic Index: Romaine Lettuce: Low (GI = 2-5) | Cherry Tomatoes: Low (GI = 15) | Cucumber: Low (GI = 15) | Red Onion: Low (GI = 10) | Kalamata Olives: Low (GI = 15) | Feta Cheese: Low (GI = 15)

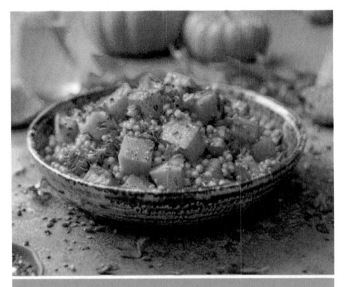

Buckwheat and Roasted Pumpkin Salad

Prep: 15 mins | Cook: 30 mins | Serves: 4

Ingredients:

- 1 cup buckwheat groats (200g)
- 2 cups diced pumpkin (300g)
- 1 red bell pepper, diced (150g)
- 1/4 cup chopped fresh parsley (15g)
- 2 tbsp olive oil (30ml)
- 1 tbsp apple cider vinegar (15ml)
- 1 tbsp low carb sweeteners
- 1 tsp salt (5g)
- 1/2 tsp black pepper (2.5g)

Instructions:

1. Preheat the oven to 400°F (200°C).
2. Cook buckwheat groats according to package instructions, then set aside to cool.
3. Toss diced pumpkin and red bell pepper with 1 tbsp olive oil, 1/2 tsp salt, and 1/4 tsp black pepper. Spread on a baking sheet and roast for 25-30 minutes until tender.
4. In a large bowl, combine cooked buckwheat, roasted pumpkin, red bell pepper, and parsley.
5. In a small bowl, whisk together remaining olive oil, apple cider vinegar, low carb sweeteners, remaining salt, and pepper to make the dressing.
6. Pour the dressing over the salad and toss to combine. Serve warm or at room temperature.

Nutritional Facts (Per Serving): Calories: 350 | Sugars: 6g | Fat: 14g | Carbohydrates: 45g | Protein: 18g | Fiber: 7g | Sodium: 480mg

Glycemic Index: Buckwheat: Medium (GI = 54) | Pumpkin: Medium (GI = 75) | Red Bell Pepper: Low (GI = 15)

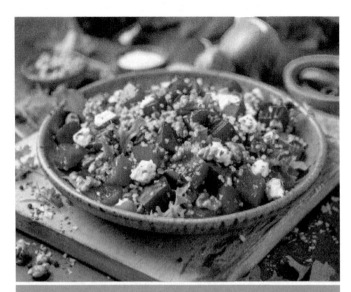

Roasted Beetroot and Quinoa Salad with Feta Cheese

Prep: 15 mins | Cook: 30 mins | Serves: 4

Ingredients:

- 1 cup quinoa (200g)
- 3 medium beetroots, diced (300g)
- 1/2 cup crumbled feta cheese (60g)
- 4 cups mixed salad greens (120g)
- 1/4 cup chopped walnuts (30g)
- 2 tbsp olive oil (30ml)
- 2 tbsp balsamic vinegar (30ml)
- 1 tbsp low carb sweeteners
- 1 tsp salt (5g)
- 1/2 tsp black pepper (2.5g)

Instructions:

1. Preheat the oven to 400°F (200°C).
2. Cook quinoa according to package instructions, then set aside to cool.
3. Toss diced beetroots with 1 tbsp olive oil, 1/2 tsp salt, and 1/4 tsp black pepper. Spread on a baking sheet and roast for 25-30 minutes until tender.
4. In a large bowl, combine cooked quinoa, roasted beetroots, crumbled feta cheese, mixed salad greens, and chopped walnuts.
5. In a small bowl, whisk together remaining olive oil, balsamic vinegar, low carb sweeteners, remaining salt, and pepper to make the dressing.
6. Pour the dressing over the salad and toss to combine. Serve chilled or at room temperature.

Nutritional Facts (Per Serving): Calories: 350 | Sugars: 6g | Fat: 15g | Carbohydrates: 45g | Protein: 18g | Fiber: 7g | Sodium: 480mg

Glycemic Index: Quinoa: Medium (GI = 53) | Beetroot: Medium (GI = 64) | Feta Cheese: Low (GI = 15) | Walnuts: Low (GI = 15)

CHAPTER 18: DINNERS: Fish And Seafood Delights

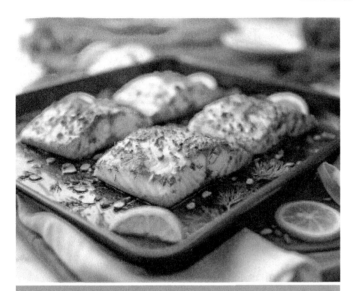

Baked Cod with Lemon and Dill

Prep: 10 mins | Cook: 20 mins | Serves: 4

Ingredients:

- 4 cod fillets (each 6 oz / 170g)
- Juice and zest of 1 lemon
- 2 tbsp chopped fresh dill (30g)
- 2 tbsp olive oil (30ml)
- 1 tsp salt (5g)
- 1/2 tsp black pepper (2.5g)
- 1/2 cup sliced almonds (60g)

Instructions:

1. Preheat the oven to 400°F (200°C).
2. Place cod fillets on a baking sheet lined with parchment paper.
3. In a small bowl, mix lemon juice, lemon zest, chopped dill, olive oil, salt, and pepper.
4. Brush the lemon and dill mixture over the cod fillets. Sprinkle sliced almonds over the top.
5. Bake for 20 minutes or until the fish is opaque and flakes easily with a fork.

Nutritional Facts (Per Serving): Calories: 350 | Sugars: 1g | Fat: 14g | Carbohydrates: 10g | Protein: 30g | Fiber: 4g | Sodium: 400mg

Glycemic Index: Cod: Negligible GI | Lemon: Negligible GI | Dill: Negligible GI | Almonds: Low (GI = 15)

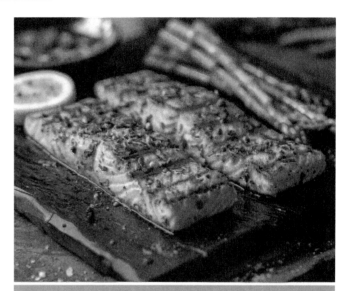

Grilled Salmon with Asparagus

Prep: 15 mins | Cook: 20 mins | Serves: 4

Ingredients:

- 4 salmon fillets (each 6 oz / 170g)
- Juice and zest of 1 lemon
- 1 lb asparagus, trimmed (450g)
- 2 tbsp olive oil (30ml)
- 1 tbsp fresh rosemary, chopped (15g)
- 1 tsp salt (5g)
- 1/2 tsp black pepper (2.5g)

Instructions:

1. Preheat the grill to medium-high heat.
2. Marinate salmon fillets in lemon juice, lemon zest, olive oil, chopped rosemary, salt, and pepper for 10 minutes.
3. Grill salmon over medium heat until cooked through, about 4-5 minutes per side.
4. Toss asparagus with olive oil, salt, and pepper.
5. Grill asparagus for 5-7 minutes, turning occasionally, until tender and slightly charred.
6. Serve the grilled salmon with asparagus.

Nutritional Facts (Per Serving): Calories: 350 | Sugars: 2g | Fat: 14g | Carbohydrates: 12g | Protein: 32g | Fiber: 6g | Sodium: 480mg

Glycemic Index: Salmon: Negligible GI | Asparagus: Low (GI = 15) | Lemon: Negligible GI | Rosemary: Negligible GI

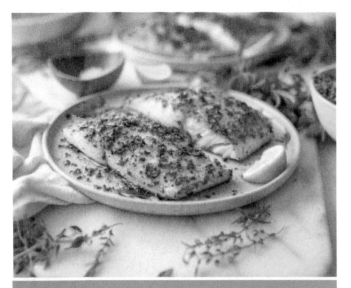

Herb-Crusted Tilapia

Prep: 10 mins | Cook: 15 mins | Serves: 4

Ingredients:

- 4 tilapia fillets (each 6 oz / 170g)
- 1/2 cup whole wheat breadcrumbs (60g)
- 1/4 cup grated Parmesan cheese (30g)
- 2 tbsp chopped fresh parsley (30g)
- 2 tbsp olive oil (30ml)
- 1 tsp dried thyme (5g)
- 1 tsp salt (5g)
- 1/2 tsp black pepper (2.5g)

Instructions:

1. Preheat the oven to 400°F (200°C).
2. In a bowl, combine breadcrumbs, grated Parmesan cheese, chopped parsley, dried thyme, salt, and pepper.
3. Brush tilapia fillets with olive oil and coat with the breadcrumb mixture.
4. Place the fillets on a baking sheet lined with parchment paper.
5. Bake for 15 minutes or until the fish is golden brown and flakes easily with a fork.

Nutritional Facts (Per Serving): Calories: 350 | Sugars: 1g | Fat: 14g | Carbohydrates: 35g | Protein: 23g | Fiber: 6g | Sodium: 470mg

Glycemic Index: Tilapia: Negligible GI | Whole Wheat Breadcrumbs: Medium (GI = 50) | Parmesan Cheese: Low (GI = 27)

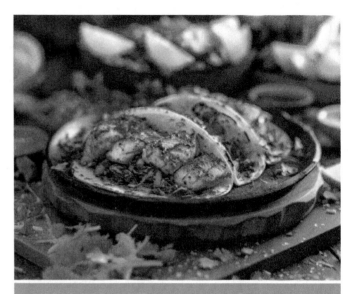

Mahi Mahi Tacos with Cabbage Slaw

Prep: 20 mins | Cook: 10 mins | Serves: 4

Ingredients:

- 4 mahi mahi fillets (each 6 oz / 170g)
- 8 small corn tortillas (200g)
- 2 cups shredded cabbage (150g)
- 1/4 cup grated carrots (30g)
- 1/4 cup Greek yogurt (60g)
- 1 tsp ground cumin (5g)
- 1 tsp salt (5g)
- 2 tbsp lime juice (30ml)
- 1 tbsp low carb sweeteners
- 1/2 tsp black pepper (2.5g)
- 1 tbsp olive oil (15ml)
- 1/4 cup chopped fresh cilantro (15g)

Instructions:

1. Preheat grill to medium-high heat.
2. Make slaw: Combine cabbage, carrots, Greek yogurt, lime juice, sweetener, and half the salt and pepper in a bowl; toss and set aside.
3. Season fish: Brush mahi mahi with olive oil; season with cumin and remaining salt and pepper.
4. Grill fish: Cook for 4–5 minutes per side until cooked through and slightly charred.
5. Warm tortillas: Grill for about 1 minute per side. Assemble tacos: Place grilled fish on tortillas, top with slaw, and garnish with cilantro.

Nutritional Facts (Per Serving): Calories: 350 | Sugars: 5g | Fat: 14g | Carbohydrates: 40g | Protein: 20g | Fiber: 7g | Sodium: 480mg

Glycemic Index: Mahi Mahi: Negligible GI | Corn Tortillas: Medium (GI = 52) | Cabbage: Low (GI = 10) | Greek Yogurt: Low (GI = 35) | Carrots: Medium (GI = 35)

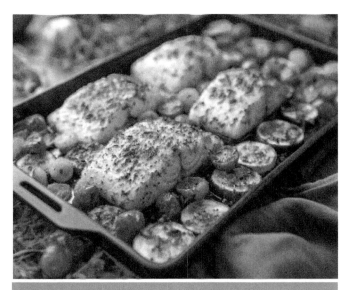

Baked Halibut with Roasted Vegetables

Prep: 15 mins | Cook: 30 mins | Serves: 4

Ingredients:

- 4 halibut fillets (each 6 oz / 170g)
- 1 red bell pepper, diced (150g)
- 1 zucchini, sliced (200g)
- 1 cup cherry tomatoes, halved (150g)
- 1 red onion, sliced (150g)
- 2 tbsp olive oil (30ml)
- 1 tsp dried oregano (5g)
- 1 tsp salt (5g)
- 1/2 tsp black pepper (2.5g)
- Juice of 1 lemon

Instructions:

1. Preheat the oven to 400°F (200°C).
2. In a large bowl, toss diced red bell pepper, sliced zucchini, cherry tomatoes, and sliced red onion with olive oil, dried oregano, salt, and black pepper.
3. Spread the vegetables on a baking sheet and place the halibut fillets on top.
4. Drizzle lemon juice over the halibut and vegetables.
5. Bake for 25-30 minutes or until the fish is opaque and flakes easily with a fork.

Nutritional Facts (Per Serving): Calories: 350 | Sugars: 6g | Fat: 14g | Carbohydrates: 35g | Protein: 23g | Fiber: 7g | Sodium: 470mg

Glycemic Index: Halibut: Negligible GI | Red Bell Pepper: Low (GI = 15) | Zucchini: Low (GI = 15) | Cherry Tomatoes: Low (GI = 15) | Red Onion: Low (GI = 10)

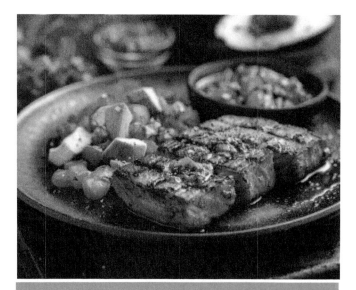

Grilled Tuna Steaks with Avocado Salsa

Prep: 15 mins | Cook: 10 mins | Serves: 4

Ingredients:

- 4 tuna steaks (each 6 oz / 170g)
- 2 tbsp olive oil (30ml)
- 1 tsp salt (5g)
- 1/2 tsp black pepper (2.5g)
- Juice of 1 lime
- 1 avocado, diced (150g)
- 1/2 cup cherry tomatoes, halved (75g)
- 1/4 cup red onion, finely chopped (35g)
- 1/4 cup fresh cilantro, chopped (15g)
- 1 tsp low carb sweeteners

Instructions:

1. Preheat the grill to medium-high heat.
2. Brush tuna steaks with olive oil and season with salt and black pepper.
3. Grill tuna steaks for 4-5 minutes per side, until desired doneness.
4. In a bowl, combine diced avocado, cherry tomatoes, chopped red onion, fresh cilantro, lime juice, and low carb sweeteners to make the avocado salsa.
5. Serve grilled tuna steaks topped with avocado salsa.

Nutritional Facts (Per Serving): Calories: 350 | Sugars: 4g | Fat: 15g | Carbohydrates: 20g | Protein: 30g | Fiber: 7g | Sodium: 480mg

Glycemic Index: Tuna: Negligible GI | Avocado: Low (GI = 15) | Cherry Tomatoes: Low (GI = 15) | Red Onion: Low (GI = 10) | Lime: Negligible GI

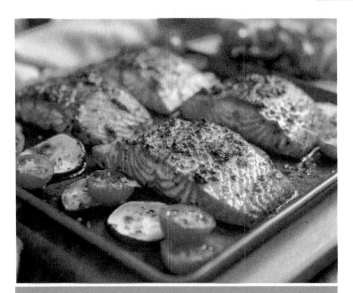

Pesto-Crusted Salmon with Vegetables

Prep: 15 mins | Cook: 20 mins | Serves: 4

Ingredients:

- 4 salmon fillets (each 6 oz / 170g)
- 1/2 cup prepared pesto (120g)
- 1 zucchini, sliced (200g)
- 1 bell pepper, sliced (150g)
- 1 cup cherry tomatoes, halved (150g)
- 2 tbsp olive oil (30ml)
- 1 tsp salt (5g)
- 1/2 tsp black pepper (2.5g)

Instructions:

1. Preheat the oven to 400°F (200°C).
2. Place salmon fillets on a baking sheet lined with parchment paper.
3. Spread 2 tbsp pesto evenly over each fillet.
4. In a large bowl, toss sliced zucchini, bell pepper, and cherry tomatoes with olive oil, salt, and pepper.
5. Arrange the vegetables around the salmon on the baking sheet.
6. Bake for 20 minutes or until the salmon is cooked through and vegetables are tender.

Nutritional Facts (Per Serving): Calories: 350 | Sugars: 6g | Fat: 15g | Carbohydrates: 35g | Protein: 22g | Fiber: 7g | Sodium: 480mg
Glycemic Index: Salmon: Negligible GI | Pesto: Low (GI = 15) | Zucchini: Low (GI = 15) | Bell Pepper: Low (GI = 15) | Cherry Tomatoes: Low (GI = 15)

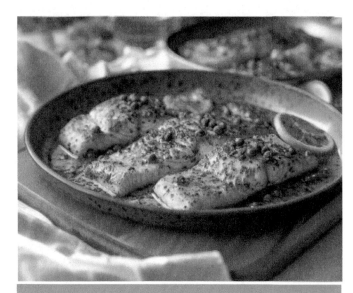

Baked Sole with Lemon and Capers

Prep: 10 mins | Cook: 15 mins | Serves: 4

Ingredients:

- 4 sole fillets (each 6 oz / 170g)
- Juice of 1 lemon
- 2 tbsp capers (30g)
- 2 tbsp olive oil (30ml)
- 1/4 cup fresh parsley, chopped (15g)
- 1 tsp salt (5g)
- 1/2 tsp black pepper (2.5g)

Instructions:

1. Preheat the oven to 375°F (190°C).
2. Place sole fillets in a baking dish.
3. Drizzle with lemon juice and olive oil.
4. Sprinkle capers, chopped parsley, salt, and black pepper over the fillets.
5. Bake for 15 minutes or until the fish is opaque and flakes easily with a fork.

Nutritional Facts (Per Serving): Calories: 350 | Sugars: 1g | Fat: 14g | Carbohydrates: 8g | Protein: 23g | Fiber: 2g | Sodium: 480mg

Glycemic Index: Sole: Negligible GI | Lemon: Negligible GI | Capers: Low (GI = 15) | Parsley: Negligible GI

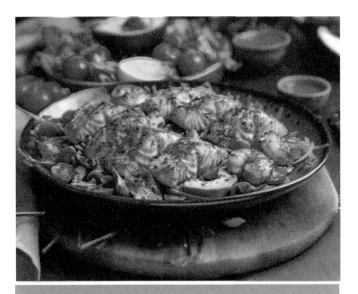

Salmon, Shrimp and Avocado Salad

Prep: 20 mins | Cook: 10 mins | Serves: 4

Ingredients:

- 2 salmon fillets (6 oz each / 170g each)
- 8 oz cooked shrimp (225g)
- 1 avocado, diced (150g)
- 4 cups mixed salad greens (120g)
- 1/2 cup cherry tomatoes, halved (75g)
- 1/4 cup red onion, thinly sliced (35g)
- 2 tbsp olive oil (30ml)
- 1 tbsp lemon juice (15ml)
- 1 tsp low carb sweeteners
- 1 tsp salt (5g)
- 1/2 tsp black pepper (2.5g)

Instructions:

1. Preheat the grill to medium-high heat.
2. Season salmon fillets with salt and black pepper. Grill for 4-5 minutes per side, until cooked through. Let cool and cut into pieces.
3. In a large bowl, combine mixed salad greens, diced avocado, cherry tomatoes, red onion, and cooked shrimp.
4. In a small bowl, whisk together olive oil, lemon juice, low carb sweeteners, remaining salt, and black pepper to make the dressing.
5. Add salmon to the salad. Drizzle with the dressing and toss to combine.

Nutritional Facts (Per Serving): Calories: 350 | Sugars: 4g | Fat: 15g | Carbohydrates: 20g | Protein: 30g | Fiber: 7g | Sodium: 480mg

Glycemic Index: Salmon: Negligible GI | Shrimp: Negligible GI | Avocado: Low (GI = 15) | Cherry Tomatoes: Low (GI = 15) | Red Onion: Low (GI = 10) | Lemon: Negligible GI

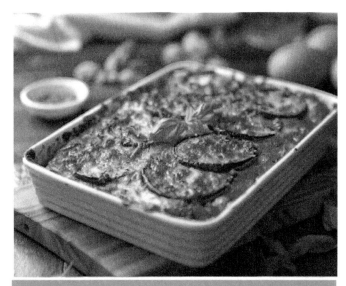

Eggplant Lasagna with Ricotta

Prep: 20 mins | Cook: 40 mins | Serves: 4

Ingredients:

- 2 large eggplants, sliced (600g)
- 1 cup ricotta cheese (240g)
- 1 cup marinara sauce (240ml)
- 1 cup shredded mozzarella cheese (120g)
- 1/2 cup grated Parmesan cheese (50g)
- 1 egg (50g)
- 2 cloves garlic, minced
- 2 tbsp olive oil (30ml)
- 1 tsp dried basil (5g)
- 1 tsp dried oregano (5g)
- 1 tsp salt (5g)
- 1/2 tsp black pepper (2.5g)

Instructions:

1. Preheat the oven to 375°F (190°C).
2. Brush eggplant slices with olive oil and season with salt and pepper. Roast on a baking sheet for 20 minutes until tender.
3. In a bowl, mix ricotta cheese, egg, minced garlic, dried basil, dried oregano, salt, and black pepper.
4. In a baking dish, layer roasted eggplant slices, ricotta mixture, marinara sauce, and shredded mozzarella cheese. Repeat the layers, finishing with a layer of mozzarella and Parmesan cheese.
5. Bake for 20 minutes until the cheese is melted and bubbly.

Nutritional Facts (Per Serving): Calories: 350 | Sugars: 6g | Fat: 15g | Carbohydrates: 35g | Protein: 20g | Fiber: 7g | Sodium: 480mg

Glycemic Index: Eggplant: Low (GI = 15) | Ricotta Cheese: Low (GI = 27) | Marinara Sauce: Medium (GI = 45) | Mozzarella Cheese: Low (GI = 32) | Parmesan Cheese: Low (GI = 27)

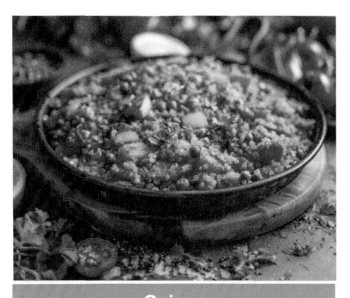

Quinoa Paella

Prep: 15 mins | Cook: 30 mins | Serves: 4

Ingredients:

- 1 cup quinoa (200g)
- 1 red, yellow bell pepper, diced (150g each)
- 1 cup green peas and cherry tomatoes, halved (150g each)
- 1/2 cup diced onion (75g)
- 3 cloves garlic, minced (9g)
- 2 cups vegetable broth (480ml)
- 2 tbsp olive oil (30ml)
- 1 tsp smoked paprika, turmeric, salt (5g each)
- 1/2 tsp black pepper (2.5g)
- 1/4 cup fresh parsley, chopped (15g)
- Juice of 1 lemon

Instructions:

1. Rinse quinoa under cold water.
2. Heat olive oil in a large pan over medium heat. Sauté diced onion and minced garlic until soft.
3. Add quinoa, diced bell peppers, green peas, and cherry tomatoes. Stir in smoked paprika, turmeric, salt, and black pepper.
4. Pour in vegetable broth, bring to a boil, then reduce heat and simmer for 20 minutes or until quinoa is cooked and liquid is absorbed.
5. Stir in fresh parsley and lemon juice before serving.

Nutritional Facts (Per Serving): Calories: 350 | Sugars: 6g | Fat: 14g | Carbohydrates: 45g | Protein: 18g | Fiber: 7g | Sodium: 480mg

Glycemic Index: Quinoa: Medium (GI = 53) | Bell Peppers: Low (GI = 15) | Green Peas: Medium (GI = 51) | Cherry Tomatoes: Low (GI = 15)

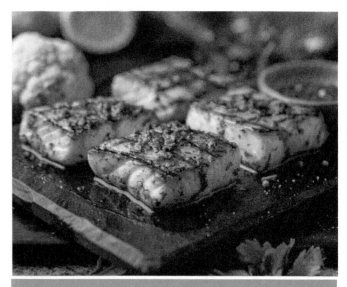

Grilled Swordfish with Herb Butter and Cauliflower

Prep: 15 mins | Cook: 20 mins | Serves: 4

Ingredients:

- 4 swordfish steaks (each 6 oz / 170g)
- 1 head cauliflower, cut into florets (600g)
- 2 tbsp olive oil (30ml)
- 1/4 cup unsalted butter (60g)
- 2 tbsp fresh parsley, chopped (15g)
- 2 tbsp fresh chives, chopped (15g)
- 1 tbsp lemon juice (15ml)
- 1 tsp salt (5g)
- 1/2 tsp black pepper (2.5g)

Instructions:

1. Preheat the grill to medium-high heat.
2. Brush swordfish steaks and cauliflower florets with olive oil and season with salt and black pepper.
3. Grill swordfish steaks for 4-5 minutes per side until cooked through. Grill cauliflower florets for 10-12 minutes until tender and slightly charred.
4. In a small saucepan, melt unsalted butter. Stir in chopped parsley, chives, and lemon juice.
5. Drizzle herb butter over grilled swordfish.

Nutritional Facts (Per Serving): Calories: 350 | Sugars: 4g | Fat: 15g | Carbohydrates: 20g | Protein: 30g | Fiber: 6g | Sodium: 480mg

Glycemic Index: Swordfish: Negligible GI | Cauliflower: Low (GI = 15) | Butter: Low (GI = 0) | Herbs: Negligible GI

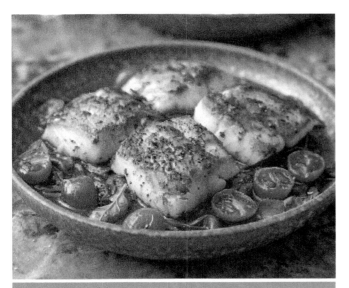

Braised Cod with Tomatoes and Spinach

Prep: 15 mins | Cook: 20 mins | Serves: 4

Ingredients:

- 4 cod fillets (each 6 oz / 170g)
- 2 cups cherry tomatoes, halved (300g)
- 4 cups fresh spinach (120g)
- 1 onion, finely chopped (150g)
- 3 cloves garlic, minced (9g)
- 1/4 cup vegetable broth (60ml)
- 2 tbsp olive oil (30ml)
- 1 tbsp lemon juice (15ml)
- 1 tsp salt (5g)
- 1/2 tsp black pepper (2.5g)

Instructions:

1. Heat olive oil in a large pan over medium heat. Sauté chopped onion and minced garlic until soft.
2. Add cherry tomatoes and cook until they start to break down.
3. Pour in vegetable broth and bring to a simmer.
4. Place cod fillets in the pan and season with salt and black pepper. Cover and cook for 10 minutes, or until the fish is opaque and flakes easily.
5. Add fresh spinach and cook until wilted.
6. Drizzle with lemon juice before serving.

Nutritional Facts (Per Serving): Calories: 350 | Sugars: 6g | Fat: 14g | Carbohydrates: 25g | Protein: 30g | Fiber: 6g | Sodium: 450mg

Glycemic Index: Cod: Negligible GI | Cherry Tomatoes: Low (GI = 15) | Spinach: Low (GI = 15) | Onion: Low (GI = 10)

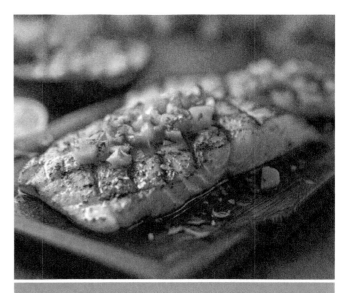

Tilapia with Mango Salsa

Prep: 15 mins | Cook: 10 mins | Serves: 4

Ingredients:

- 4 tilapia fillets (each 6 oz / 170g)
- 1 ripe mango, diced (200g)
- 1 red bell pepper, diced (150g)
- 1/4 cup red onion, finely chopped (35g)
- 1/4 cup fresh cilantro, chopped (15g)
- 1 tbsp lime juice (15ml)
- 1 tbsp olive oil (15ml)
- 1 tsp salt (5g)
- 1/2 tsp black pepper (2.5g)

Instructions:

1. Preheat the grill to medium-high heat.
2. Brush tilapia fillets with olive oil and season with salt and black pepper.
3. Grill tilapia for 4-5 minutes per side, until cooked through.
4. In a bowl, combine diced mango, red bell pepper, red onion, fresh cilantro, and lime juice to make the mango salsa.
5. Serve grilled tilapia topped with mango salsa.

Nutritional Facts (Per Serving): Calories: 350 | Sugars: 7g | Fat: 12g | Carbohydrates: 35g | Protein: 23g | Fiber: 7g | Sodium: 480mg

Glycemic Index: Tilapia: Negligible GI | Mango: Medium (GI = 55) | Red Bell Pepper: Low (GI = 15) | Red Onion: Low (GI = 10) | Lime: Negligible G

CHAPTER 20: BONUSES

Meal Planning and Shopping Templates

We've created a 30-day grocery shopping guide aligned with the recipes in this cookbook to make your diabetic meal planning easier. Designed for one person, this guide focuses on fresh, whole foods while minimizing processed items. Be mindful of hidden sugars, especially in sauces and dressings. Adjust quantities as needed to fit your dietary preferences. Enjoy cooking healthy, flavorful meals that support your blood sugar management!

Grocery Shopping List for 7-Day Meal Plan

Meat & Poultry:

- **Chicken breast (boneless, skinless)** – 1 lb / 450 g *(Grilled Chicken and Veggie Bowl, Wild Rice Burrito)*
- **Ground turkey** – 1 lb / 450 g *(Ground Turkey and Vegetable Casserole)*
- **Beef stew meat** – 1 lb / 450 g *(Beef and Barley Stew)*
- **Turkey slices** – 4 oz / 115 g *(Turkey and Cheese Roll-ups)*
- **Eggs** – 18 large *(Zucchini and Cheese Frittata, Veggie Egg Muffins, Various Recipes)*

Fish & Seafood:

- **Salmon fillets** – 1.5 lb / 680 g *(Grilled Salmon with Asparagus, Pesto-Crusted Salmon)*
- **Cod fillets** – 1 lb / 450 g *(Baked Cod with Lemon and Dill, Braised Cod with Tomatoes and Spinach)*
- **Tuna steaks** – 2 steaks (about 12 oz / 340 g) *(Grilled Tuna Steaks with Avocado Salsa)*
- **Tilapia fillets** – 2 fillets (about 8 oz / 225 g) *(Herb-Crusted Tilapia)*

Vegetables:

- **Spinach (fresh)** – 10 cups / 300 g *(Spinach Smoothie, Chickpea and Spinach Curry, Braised Cod)*
- **Zucchini** – 4 medium *(Zucchini Frittata, Veggie Egg Muffins, Stuffed Mushrooms)*
- **Eggplant** – 2 large *(Eggplant Lasagna, Eggplant Rolls)*
- **Cauliflower florets** – 2 cups / 300 g *(Wild Rice Burrito)*
- **Asparagus** – 1 bunch *(Grilled Salmon with Asparagus)*
- **Bell peppers** – 3 medium *(Ground Turkey Casserole, Grilled Chicken Bowl, Quinoa Salad)*
- **Cucumbers** – 2 medium *(Cucumber Slices with Hummus, Greek Yogurt with Cucumbers)*
- **Tomatoes** – 4 medium *(Braised Cod, Eggplant Lasagna)*
- **Onions** – 6 medium *(Various Recipes)*
- **Garlic** – 1 bulb
- **Mushrooms** – 8 oz / 225 g *(Stuffed Mushrooms)*
- **Avocados** – 4 large *(Spinach Smoothie, Quinoa Salad, Tuna Steaks, Wild Rice Burrito)*
- **Carrots** – 3 medium *(Beef Stew, Ground Turkey Casserole)*
- **Fresh herbs** (parsley, dill, basil) – 1 bunch each
- **Baby spinach** – included in spinach quantity *(Braised Cod with Tomatoes and Spinach)*

Fruits:

- **Bananas** – 2 medium *(Almond Butter and Banana Smoothie)*
- **Blueberries** – 1 cup / 150 g *(Almond Flour Blueberry Muffins, Cottage Cheese Breakfast)*
- **Lemons** – 3 medium *(Baked Cod, Herb-Crusted Tilapia, Pesto Salmon)*
- **Limes** – 2 medium *(Tuna Steaks with Avocado Salsa)*

Grains & Legumes:

- **Quinoa** – 1 cup / 180 g *(Quinoa and Black Bean Salad)*
- **Farro** – 1 cup / 200 g *(Farro and Roasted Vegetable Bowl)*
- **Barley** – 1 cup / 200 g *(Beef and Barley Stew)*
- **Wild rice** – 1 cup / 185 g *(Wild Rice Burrito)*
- **Black beans** (canned) – 1 can (15 oz / 425 g) *(Quinoa and Black Bean Salad)*
- **Chickpeas** (canned) – 1 can (15 oz / 425 g) *(Chickpea and Spinach Curry)*
- **Whole wheat tortillas** – 2 medium *(Wild Rice Burrito)*

Dairy & Eggs:

- **Almond milk** (unsweetened) – 2 cups / 480 ml *(Chia Seed Pudding, Almond Banana Smoothie)*
- **Almond flour** – 2 cups / 200 g *(Blueberry Muffins, Chocolate Chip Cookies)*
- **Cottage cheese** – 1 cup / 240 g *(Cottage Cheese with Almonds and Blueberries)*
- **Feta cheese** – 4 oz / 115 g *(Stuffed Mushrooms)*
- **Ricotta cheese** – 1 cup / 250 g *(Eggplant Lasagna)*
- **Cheddar cheese** (shredded) – 1 cup / 100 g *(Ground Turkey Casserole)*

- **Cream cheese** – 8 oz / 225 g (*Lemon Cheesecake Bars*)
- **Greek yogurt** (plain) – 1 cup / 240 g (*Greek Yogurt with Cucumbers*)
- **Mozzarella cheese** – 1 cup / 100 g (*Eggplant Lasagna*)
- **Parmesan cheese** – ½ cup / 50 g (*Herb-Crusted Tilapia*)

Nuts & Seeds:

- **Almonds** (sliced) – 1 cup/100 g (*Cottage Cheese Breakfast, Chia Seed Pudding*)
- **Mixed nuts** – ½ cup / 75 g (*Chia Seed Pudding*)
- **Almond butter** – ½ cup / 125 g (*Almond Butter and Banana Smoothie*)
- **Chia seeds** – ½ cup / 75 g (*Chia Seed Pudding*)

Pantry Staples:

- **Olive oil** (extra virgin) – 1 bottle (*Various Recipes*)
- **Low-carb sweetener** – 1 cup / 200 g (*Blueberry Muffins, Lemon Cheesecake Bars, Chocolate Chip Cookies*)
- **Hummus** – ½ cup / 120 g (*Cucumber Slices with Hummus*)
- **Tomato sauce** (no added sugar) – 1 cup / 240 ml (*Eggplant Lasagna, Ground Turkey Casserole*)
- **Coconut flour** – ½ cup / 60 g (*Chocolate Chip Cookies*)
- **Baking powder** – 1 small container
- **Vanilla extract** – 1 small bottle (*Cheesecake Bars, Muffins, Cookies*)
- **Dark chocolate chips** (sugar-free) – ½ cup / 85 g (*Low-Carb Chocolate Chip Cookies*)
- **Spices and herbs:** cumin, oregano, basil, rosemary, thyme, paprika, chili powder, black pepper, sea salt
- **Dijon mustard** – small jar

(*Tuna Steaks with Avocado Salsa*)
- **Soy sauce** (low-sodium) – small bottle (*Braised Cod with Tomatoes and Spinach*)
- **Balsamic vinegar** – small bottle (*Grilled Chicken and Veggie Bowl*)

Other:

- **Whole grain bread or wraps** – as needed (*Turkey and Cheese Roll-ups*)
- **Unsweetened cocoa powder** – ¼ cup / 25 g (*Chocolate Chip Cookies*)

Grocery Shopping List for 8-14 Day Meal Plan

Meat & Poultry:

- **Chicken breast (boneless, skinless)** – 2 lb / 900 g (*Chicken and Turkey Cutlets, Kale and Chicken Caesar Salad, Zucchini Noodles with Pesto Chicken, Asian-Inspired Chicken Salad*)
- **Ground turkey** – 1.5 lb / 680 g (*Chicken and Turkey Cutlets, Stuffed Cabbage Rolls, Broccoli and Turkey Meatball Lunch Box*)
- **Turkey sausage** – 0.5 lb / 225 g (*Turkey Sausage and Pepper Breakfast Bake*)
- **Eggs** – 18 large (*Zucchini and Mushroom Egg Bake, Mushroom and Swiss Cheese Omelette, Spinach and Ricotta Crepes, Turkey Sausage and Pepper Breakfast Bake, Various Recipes*)

Fish & Seafood:

- **Halibut fillets** – 1 lb / 450 g (*Baked Halibut with Roasted Vegetables*)
- **Mahi Mahi fillets** – 1 lb / 450 g (*Mahi Mahi Tacos with Cabbage Slaw*)
- **Swordfish steaks** – 1 lb / 450 g (*Grilled Swordfish with Herb*

Butter and Cauliflower*)
- **Tilapia fillets** – 1 lb / 450 g (*Tilapia with Mango Salsa*)
- **Sole fillets** – 1 lb / 450 g (*Baked Sole with Lemon and Capers*)

Vegetables:

- **Zucchini** – 6 medium (*Zucchini and Mushroom Egg Bake, Zucchini Noodles with Pesto Chicken, Broccoli and Turkey Meatball Lunch Box*)
- **Mushrooms** – 16 oz / 450 g (*Zucchini and Mushroom Egg Bake, Buckwheat Porridge, Mushroom and Swiss Cheese Omelette*)
- **Spinach (fresh)** – 3 bunches (*Spinach and Feta Stuffed Peppers, Hearty Lentil and Spinach Soup, Spinach and Ricotta Crepes, Artichoke and Spinach Yogurt Dip*)
- **Bell peppers** – 6 medium (assorted colors) (*Spinach and Feta Stuffed Peppers, Turkey Sausage and Pepper Breakfast Bake, Sliced Bell Peppers with Guacamole*)
- **Cabbage** – 1 large head (*Stuffed Cabbage Rolls, Mahi Mahi Tacos with Cabbage Slaw*)
- **Cauliflower heads** – 2 medium (*Roasted Cauliflower Steaks, Grilled Swordfish with Cauliflower*)
- **Kale** – 1 bunch (*Kale and Chicken Caesar Salad*)
- **Eggplant** – 1 large (*Artichoke and Spinach Yogurt Dip*)
- **Broccoli florets** – 2 cups / 300 g (*Broccoli and Turkey Meatball Lunch Box*)
- **Onions** – 8 medium (*Various recipes*)
- **Garlic** – 2 bulbs
- **Avocados** – 3 large (*Chicken and Avocado Salad, Asian-Inspired Chicken Salad, Guacamole*)
- **Tomatoes** – 6 medium (*Mahi Mahi Tacos, Tilapia with Mango Salsa, Asian-Inspired Chicken Salad*)
- **Lettuce leaves** – 1 head (butter

lettuce or romaine) *(Breakfast Burrito with Lettuce Wrap, Mahi Mahi Tacos)*
- **Fresh herbs** (parsley, cilantro, basil, mint) – 1 bunch each

---

Fruits:

- **Lemons** – 6 medium *(Baked Halibut, Grilled Swordfish, Baked Sole, Various recipes)*
- **Limes** – 4 medium *(Mahi Mahi Tacos, Tilapia with Mango Salsa, Guacamole)*
- **Oranges** – 2 medium *(Quinoa Breakfast Bowl)*
- **Bananas** – 1 medium *(Quinoa Breakfast Bowl)*
- **Mangoes** – 1 large *(Tilapia with Mango Salsa)*
- **Berries (raspberries)** – 1 cup / 150 g *(Almond Flour Raspberry Bars)*
- **Pumpkin puree (canned)** – 1 cup / 240 g *(Low-Carb Pumpkin Pie, Buckwheat and Roasted Pumpkin Salad)*

Grains & Bread:

- **Quinoa** – 1 cup / 180 g *(Quinoa Breakfast Bowl, Stuffed Cabbage Rolls)*
- **Buckwheat groats** – 2 cups / 400 g *(Buckwheat Porridge, Buckwheat and Roasted Pumpkin Salad)*
- **Brown rice** – 1 cup / 200 g *(Brown Rice Pilaf)*
- **Whole wheat tortillas or lettuce leaves** – 4 large *(Breakfast Burrito with Lettuce Wrap, Mahi Mahi Tacos)*

Dairy & Eggs:

- **Swiss cheese** – 4 oz / 115 g *(Mushroom and Swiss Cheese Omelette)*
- **Feta cheese** – 8 oz / 225 g *(Spinach and Feta Stuffed Peppers, Spinach and Ricotta Crepes)*
- **Ricotta cheese** – 1 cup / 250 g

(Spinach and Ricotta Crepes)
- **Cheddar cheese (shredded)** – 1 cup / 100 g *(Zucchini and Mushroom Egg Bake)*
- **Parmesan cheese** – 4 oz / 115 g *(Kale and Chicken Caesar Salad, Zucchini Noodles with Pesto Chicken)*
- **Mozzarella cheese** – 4 oz / 115 g *(Broccoli and Turkey Meatball Lunch Box)*
- **Greek yogurt (plain)** – 2 cups / 500 g *(Artichoke and Spinach Yogurt Dip, Kale and Chicken Caesar Salad)*
- **Unsweetened almond milk** – 2 cups / 480 ml *(Vanilla Chia Seed Pudding)*
- **Heavy cream** – 1 cup / 240 ml *(Low-Carb Tiramisu)*

Nuts, Seeds & Nut Butter:

- **Almond flour** – 2 cups / 200 g *(Almond Flour Raspberry Bars, Lemon Coconut Balls)*
- **Chia seeds** – ½ cup / 75 g *(Vanilla Chia Seed Pudding)*
- **Almonds (sliced or whole)** – 1 cup / 150 g *(Quinoa Breakfast Bowl, Almond Flour Raspberry Bars)*
- **Walnuts** – ½ cup / 75 g *(Buckwheat Porridge)*
- **Coconut flakes (unsweetened)** – 1 cup / 100 g *(Lemon Coconut Balls)*
- **Cashews** – ½ cup / 75 g *(Asian-Inspired Chicken Salad)*
- **Sesame seeds** – ¼ cup / 40 g *(Asian-Inspired Chicken Salad)*

Pantry Staples:

- **Olive oil (extra virgin)** – 1 bottle *(Various recipes)*
- **Coconut oil** – ½ cup / 120 ml *(Coconut Flour Brownies, Lemon Coconut Balls)*
- **Coconut flour** – 1 cup / 120 g *(Coconut Flour Brownies)*
- **Low-carb sweetener** – 1.5 cups / 300 g *(Coconut Flour Brownies, Low-Carb Tiramisu, Lemon Coconut Balls, Low-Carb Pumpkin Pie)*

- **Cocoa powder (unsweetened)** – ½ cup / 50 g *(Coconut Flour Brownies, Low-Carb Tiramisu)*
- **Vanilla extract** – 1 small bottle *(Vanilla Chia Seed Pudding, Low-Carb Tiramisu, Lemon Coconut Balls)*
- **Baking powder** – 1 small container *(Almond Flour Raspberry Bars, Coconut Flour Brownies)*
- **Baking soda** – 1 small container *(Low-Carb Pumpkin Pie)*
- **Pumpkin pie spice** – 1 small jar *(Low-Carb Pumpkin Pie, Buckwheat and Roasted Pumpkin Salad)*
- **Artichoke hearts (canned)** – 1 can *(Artichoke and Spinach Yogurt Dip)*
- **Capers** – 1 small jar *(Baked Sole with Lemon and Capers)*
- **Mustard (Dijon)** – 1 small jar *(Kale and Chicken Caesar Salad, Chicken and Turkey Cutlets)*
- **Soy sauce (low-sodium)** – 1 bottle *(Asian-Inspired Chicken Salad)*
- **Sesame oil** – 1 small bottle *(Asian-Inspired Chicken Salad)*
- **Balsamic vinegar** – 1 small bottle *(Various recipes)*
- **Pesto sauce** – 1 jar or ingredients to make homemade pesto *(Zucchini Noodles with Pesto Chicken)*
- **Spices and herbs:** *(Salt and black pepper, Paprika, Cumin, Chili powder, Cinnamon, Nutmeg, Oregano, Thyme, Rosemary, Turmeric, Ground ginger)*

Other:

- **Guacamole or ingredients to make it** (avocados, lime, cilantro) *(Sliced Bell Peppers with Guacamole)*
- **Whole grain mustard** – small jar *(Chicken and Turkey Cutlets)*
- **Dark chocolate (85% cocoa or higher)** – 4 oz / 115 g *(Low-Carb Tiramisu)*
- **Coconut cream** – 1 can

(Low-Carb Tiramisu)

Grocery Shopping List for 15-21 Day Meal Plan

Meat & Poultry:

- **Chicken breast (boneless, skinless)** – 2 lb / 900 g *(Chicken and Spinach Breakfast Wrap, Quinoa Paella, Salmon, Shrimp, and Avocado Salad)*
- **Ground beef or turkey** – 1 lb / 450 g *(Meatballs with Couscous, Low-Carb Breakfast Casserole)*
- **Sausage or bacon** – 8 oz / 225 g *(Low-Carb Breakfast Casserole)*
- **Beef stew meat** – 1 lb / 450 g *(Beef and Barley Stew)*

Fish & Seafood:

- **Sole fillets** – 1 lb / 450 g *(Baked Sole with Lemon and Capers)*
- **Tilapia fillets** – 1 lb / 450 g *(Herb-Crusted Tilapia)*
- **Salmon fillet** – 8 oz / 225 g *(Salmon, Shrimp, and Avocado Salad)*
- **Shrimp (peeled and deveined)** – 12 oz / 340 g *(Quinoa Paella, Salmon, Shrimp, and Avocado Salad)*
- **Cod fillets** – 1 lb / 450 g *(Baked Cod with Lemon and Dill)*

Vegetables:

- **Spinach (fresh)** – 4 bunches / 1 lb / 450 g *(Spinach and Ricotta Crepes, Hearty Lentil Soup, Artichoke Dip, Warm Lentil Salad, Avocado and Spinach Omelette, Chicken and Spinach Wrap, Stuffed Acorn Squash)*
- **Zucchini** – 4 medium *(Zucchini Fritters, Warm Lentil Salad, Roasted Veggie Wrap)*
- **Eggplant** – 3 medium *(Artichoke and Spinach Yogurt Dip, Eggplant and Lentil Salad)*
- **Bell peppers** – 6 medium (assorted colors) *(Meatballs with Couscous, Grilled Green Beans and Mushrooms, Roasted Veggie Wrap, Quinoa Paella)*
- **Mushrooms** – 16 oz / 450 g *(Buckwheat Porridge, Grilled Green Beans and Mushrooms, Low-Carb Breakfast Casserole)*
- **Green beans** – 1 lb / 450 g *(Grilled Green Beans with Lemon Zest and Mushrooms)*
- **Onions** – 8 medium
- **Garlic** – 2 bulbs *(Various recipes)*
- **Carrots** – 6 medium *(Hearty Lentil Soup, Beef and Barley Stew, Carrot and Ginger Smoothie)*
- **Celery stalks** – 4 stalks *(Hearty Lentil Soup, Beef and Barley Stew)*
- **Avocados** – 5 large *(Avocado and Spinach Omelette, Chocolate Avocado Pudding, Salmon, Shrimp, and Avocado Salad)*
- **Tomatoes** – 6 medium *(Quinoa Paella, Eggplant and Lentil Salad)*
- **Cucumbers** – 2 medium *(Greek Yogurt with Cucumbers, Salmon Salad)*
- **Acorn squash** – 2 medium *(Chickpea and Spinach Stuffed Acorn Squash)*
- **Lemons** – 6 medium *(Baked Sole, Herb-Crusted Tilapia, Baked Cod, Salad Dressings)*
- **Limes** – 2 medium *(Salmon Salad Dressing)*
- **Fresh herbs** (parsley, dill, mint, basil) – 1 bunch each *(Various recipes)*
- **Baby spinach or mixed greens** – 4 cups / 120 g *(Salads, Wraps)*
- **Kale or arugula** – 1 bunch *(Warm Lentil Salad, Farro Bowl)*
- **Eggplant** – already listed
- **Ginger root** – 1 small piece *(Carrot and Ginger Smoothie)*
- **Green onions** – 1 bunch *(Zucchini Fritters)*

Fruits:

- **Bananas** – 2 medium *(Low-Carb Banana Nut Muffins)*
- **Raspberries** – 1 cup / 150 g *(Raspberry Almond Tarts)*
- **Oranges** – 2 medium *(Carrot and Ginger Smoothie, Quinoa Paella)*
- **Apples** – 1 medium

Grains & Legumes:

- **Almond flour** – 3 cups / 300 g *(Keto Pancakes, Banana Nut Muffins, Snickerdoodle Cookies)*
- **Coconut flour** – 1 cup / 120 g *(Keto Pancakes, Banana Nut Muffins)*
- **Quinoa** – 1 cup / 180 g *(Quinoa Paella)*
- **Couscous (whole wheat preferred)** – 1 cup / 180 g *(Meatballs with Couscous)*
- **Barley** – 1 cup / 200 g *(Beef and Barley Stew)*
- **Farro** – 1 cup / 200 g *(Farro and Roasted Vegetable Bowl)*
- **Lentils** – 2 cups / 400 g *(Hearty Lentil Soup, Warm Lentil Salad, Eggplant and Lentil Salad)*
- **Buckwheat groats** – 1 cup / 200 g *(Buckwheat Porridge)*
- **Chickpeas (canned or dried)** – 1 can / 15 oz / 425 g *(Stuffed Acorn Squash)*
- **Whole wheat tortillas or lettuce leaves** – 4 large *(Roasted Veggie Wrap, Chicken and Spinach Breakfast Wrap)*
- **Low-carb sweetener** (e.g., stevia, erythritol) – 1.5 cups / 300 g *(Keto Pancakes, Muffins, Cookies, Pudding, Tarts)*

Dairy & Eggs:

- **Eggs** – 2 dozen / 24 large *(Various recipes)*
- **Ricotta cheese** – 1 cup / 250 g *(Spinach and Ricotta Crepes)*
- **Cream cheese** – 8 oz / 225 g *(Keto Pancakes)*
- **Greek yogurt (plain, unsweetened)** – 2 cups / 500 g *(Artichoke and Spinach Yogurt Dip, Greek Yogurt with*

Cucumbers, Mint Yogurt Dressing)
- **Cheddar cheese (shredded)** – 1 cup / 100 g *(Low-Carb Breakfast Casserole)*
- **Mozzarella cheese** – 1 cup / 100 g *(Low-Carb Breakfast Casserole)*
- **Feta cheese** – 8 oz / 225 g *(Warm Lentil Salad, Farro Bowl)*
- **Parmesan cheese** – 4 oz / 115 g *(Zucchini Fritters, Farro Bowl)*
- **Sour cream** – 1 cup / 240 g *(Zucchini Fritters)*
- **Unsweetened almond milk** – 4 cups / 1 L *(Keto Pancakes, Smoothie, Chocolate Avocado Pudding)*
- **Butter** – 1 stick / 4 oz / 113 g *(Various recipes)*

Nuts, Seeds & Nut Butter:

- **Almonds (whole or sliced)** – 1.5 cups / 225 g *(Vanilla Almond Protein Bars, Raspberry Almond Tarts)*
- **Walnuts or pecans** – 1 cup / 150 g *(Banana Nut Muffins, Warm Lentil Salad)*
- **Almond butter** – 1 cup / 250 g *(Vanilla Almond Protein Bars)*
- **Chia seeds** – ½ cup / 75 g *(Optional for smoothies or toppings)*
- **Flaxseeds (ground)** – ½ cup / 75 g *(Optional for added fiber)*
- **Pumpkin seeds** – ½ cup / 75 g *(Warm Lentil Salad)*
- **Protein powder (vanilla, optional)** – ½ cup / 60 g *(Vanilla Almond Protein Bars)*

Pantry Staples:

- **Olive oil (extra virgin)** – 1 bottle
- **Coconut oil** – 1 cup / 240 ml *(Keto Pancakes, Muffins, Protein Bars, Tarts)*
- **Baking powder** – 1 small container *(Keto Pancakes, Muffins, Cookies)*
- **Baking soda** – 1 small container *(Banana Nut Muffins)*
- **Vanilla extract** – 1 small bottle
- **Cinnamon** – 1 small jar

(Banana Nut Muffins, Snickerdoodle Cookies)
- **Unsweetened cocoa powder** – ½ cup / 50 g *(Chocolate Avocado Pudding, Snickerdoodle Cookies)*
- **Tomato sauce or diced tomatoes (no added sugar)** – 2 cans / 14 oz / 400 g each *(Hearty Lentil Soup, Beef and Barley Stew, Quinoa Paella)*
- **Capers** – 1 small jar *(Baked Sole with Lemon and Capers)*
- **Artichoke hearts (canned)** – 1 can / 14 oz / 400 g *(Artichoke and Spinach Yogurt Dip)*
- **Hummus** – 1 cup / 240 g *(Roasted Veggie and Hummus Wrap)*
- **Mustard (Dijon)** – small jar

Spices & Herbs:

- **Dried herbs:** thyme, oregano, basil, rosemary, bay leaves
- **Spices:** cumin, paprika, chili powder, turmeric, ginger powder
- **Salt and black pepper**

> **Grocery Shopping List for 22-28 Day Meal Plan**

Meat & Poultry:

- **Chicken breast (boneless, skinless)** – 2 lb / 900 g *(Spinach and Grilled Chicken Salad, Grilled Chicken and Veggie Bowl, Zucchini Noodles with Pesto Chicken, Chicken and Avocado Salad)*
- **Ground turkey** – 1.5 lb / 680 g *(Turkey Meatloaf with Spinach and Roasted Vegetables, Stuffed Cabbage Rolls, Broccoli and Turkey Meatballs)*
- **Ham (diced, lean, low-sodium)** – 8 oz / 225 g *(Cauliflower and Ham Breakfast Casserole)*
- **Bacon** – 8 slices *(Bacon and Avocado Salad, Keto Breakfast Pizza)*
- **Eggs** – 2 dozen / 24 large *(Oatmeal Topping, Muffins, Waffles, Breakfast Casserole, Egg Bake,*

Lemon Pound Cake, Various Recipes)

Fish & Seafood:

- **Salmon fillets** – 1.5 lb / 680 g *(Grilled Salmon with Asparagus, Pesto-Crusted Salmon, Smoked Salmon for Waffles)*
- **Tilapia fillets** – 1 lb / 450 g *(Herb-Crusted Tilapia)*
- **Tuna steaks** – 2 steaks (about 12 oz / 340 g) *(Grilled Tuna Steaks with Avocado Salsa)*
- **Shrimp (peeled and deveined)** – 8 oz / 225 g

Vegetables:

- **Spinach (fresh)** – 4 bunches / 1 lb / 450 g *(Turkey Meatloaf, Grilled Chicken Salad, Orange and Spinach Smoothie, Eggplant Lasagna, Stuffed Mushrooms)*
- **Asparagus** – 2 bunches *(Grilled Salmon with Asparagus, Pesto-Crusted Salmon with Vegetables)*
- **Zucchini** – 6 medium *(Zucchini and Feta Stuffed Mushrooms, Zucchini Noodles with Pesto Chicken, Zucchini and Mushroom Egg Bake)*
- **Mushrooms** – 16 oz / 450 g *(Stuffed Mushrooms, Egg Bake, Eggplant Lasagna, Broccoli and Turkey Meatballs)*
- **Broccoli florets** – 2 cups / 300 g *(Grilled Chicken and Veggie Bowl, Broccoli and Turkey Meatballs)*
- **Bell peppers** – 6 medium (assorted colors) *(Grilled Chicken and Veggie Bowl, Sliced Bell Peppers with Guacamole, Keto Breakfast Pizza)*
- **Eggplant** – 2 large *(Eggplant Lasagna)*
- **Cauliflower heads** – 2 medium *(Cauliflower Breakfast Casserole, Pesto-Crusted Salmon with Vegetables)*
- **Cabbage leaves** – 8 large leaves *(Stuffed Cabbage Rolls)*
- **Avocados** – 6 large *(Almond Flour Waffles, Quinoa Salad, Grilled Chicken Salad, Bacon and Avocado Salad, Chicken and Avocado Salad,*

Tuna Steaks with Avocado Salsa)

- **Tomatoes** – 8 medium
(*Spinach and Grilled Chicken Salad, Eggplant Lasagna, Grilled Tuna Steaks, Broccoli and Turkey Meatballs*)
- **Onions** – 8 medium
- **Garlic** – 2 bulbs
Carrots – 4 medium (*Turkey Meatloaf, Stuffed Cabbage Rolls, Grilled Chicken and Veggie Bowl*)
- **Beetroot** – 2 medium
(*Roasted Beetroot and Quinoa Salad*)
- **Lettuce leaves** – 1 head
(*Spinach and Grilled Chicken Salad, Chicken and Avocado Salad*)
- **Cucumbers** – 2 medium
(*Sliced for salads, Sliced Bell Peppers with Guacamole*)
- **Bell peppers** – already listed
- **Fresh herbs** (parsley, basil, dill) – 1 bunch each

Fruits:

- **Bananas** – 3 medium
(*Oatmeal topping, Orange and Spinach Smoothie*)
- **Oranges** – 2 medium
(*Orange and Spinach Smoothie*)
- **Lemons** – 6 medium (*Sugar-Free Lemon Poppy Seed Muffins, Low-Carb Lemon Cheesecake Bars, Lemon Pound Cake, Herb-Crusted Tilapia, Pesto-Crusted Salmon*)
- **Avocados** – already listed

Grains & Legumes:

- **Old-fashioned oats** – 2 cups / 180 g (*Oatmeal with Bananas and Walnuts, Sugar-Free Lemon Poppy Seed Muffins*)
- **Quinoa** – 2 cups / 360 g
(*Quinoa and Black Bean Salad, Roasted Beetroot and Quinoa Salad, Stuffed Cabbage Rolls*)
- **Black beans** (canned) – 1 can (15 oz / 425 g) (*Quinoa and Black Bean Salad*)
- **Whole wheat flour** – 1 cup / 125 g (*Sugar-Free Lemon Poppy Seed Muffins*)

- **Coconut flour** – 1.5 cups / 180 g (*Coconut Flour Brownies, Low-Carb Chocolate Chip Cookies*)
- **Almond flour** – 4 cups / 400 g (*Almond Flour Waffles, Lemon Cheesecake Bars, Lemon Pound Cake*)
- **Whole wheat tortillas or wraps** – 2 large (*Grilled Chicken and Veggie Bowl, Optional for wraps*)

Dairy & Eggs:

- **Eggs** – 2 dozen / 24 large
(*Various recipes including Muffins, Waffles, Breakfast Casserole, Egg Bake, Lemon Pound Cake, Meatloaf, Cookies*)
- **Greek yogurt (plain, unsweetened)** – 2 cups / 500 g (*Low-Carb Lemon Cheesecake Bars, Guacamole, Various dressings*)
- **Ricotta cheese** – 1.5 cups / 375 g (*Eggplant Lasagna*)
- **Cream cheese** – 16 oz / 450 g (*Low-Carb Lemon Cheesecake Bars, Lemon Pound Cake*)
- **Feta cheese** – 8 oz / 225 g
(*Zucchini and Feta Stuffed Mushrooms, Roasted Beetroot and Quinoa Salad*)
- **Cheddar cheese (shredded)** – 1 cup / 100 g (*Cauliflower and Ham Breakfast Casserole, Keto Breakfast Pizza*)
- **Mozzarella cheese** – 1 cup / 100 g (*Eggplant Lasagna, Keto Breakfast Pizza*)
- **Parmesan cheese** – 4 oz / 115 g (*Grilled Chicken and Veggie Bowl, Pesto-Crusted Salmon*)
- **Milk (unsweetened almond milk or low-fat dairy milk)** – 2 cups / 480 ml (*Muffins, Waffles, Pancakes, Lemon Pound Cake*)
- **Unsalted butter** – 1 cup / 225 g (*Muffins, Cookies, Lemon Pound Cake, Various recipes*)

Nuts, Seeds & Nut Butter:

- **Walnuts** – 1 cup / 150 g
(*Oatmeal topping, Muffins, Brownies*)
- **Almonds (sliced or chopped)** – 1

cup / 150 g (*Almond Flour Waffles, Lemon Cheesecake Bars, Lemon Pound Cake*)
- **Poppy seeds** – 2 tablespoons / 30 g (*Sugar-Free Lemon Poppy Seed Muffins*)
- **Chia seeds** – ½ cup / 75 g
- **Dark chocolate chips (sugar-free)** – 1 cup / 170 g
(*Low-Carb Chocolate Chip Cookies, Coconut Flour Brownies*)

Pantry Staples:

- **Olive oil (extra virgin)** – 1 bottle
- **Coconut oil** – 1 cup / 240 ml
(*Muffins, Brownies, Cookies, Lemon Pound Cake*)
- **Baking powder** – 1 small container (*Muffins, Waffles, Pancakes, Lemon Pound Cake*)
- **Baking soda** – 1 small container (*Muffins, Brownies, Cookies, Lemon Pound Cake*)
- **Vanilla extract** – 1 small bottle (*Muffins, Waffles, Cheesecake Bars, Brownies, Cookies, Lemon Pound Cake*)
- **Low-carb sweetener** – 2 cups / 400 g
- **Unsweetened cocoa powder** – ½ cup / 50 g (*Coconut Flour Brownies*)
- **Pesto sauce** – 1 jar or ingredients to make homemade pesto (*Zucchini Noodles with Pesto Chicken, Pesto-Crusted Salmon*)
- **Tomato sauce (no added sugar)** – 1 can (14 oz / 400 g)
(*Eggplant Lasagna*)
- **Mustard (Dijon)** – small jar
- **Soy sauce (low-sodium)** – small bottle (*Grilled Tuna Steaks with Avocado Salsa*)
- **Apple cider vinegar or balsamic vinegar** – small bottle
(*Salad dressings, Quinoa Salad*)
- **Spices & Herbs:**
  - **Dried herbs:** oregano, basil, thyme, rosemary
  - **Spices:** cinnamon, nutmeg, paprika, chili powder, cumin
  - **Salt and black pepper**
- **Almond butter or peanut butter (natural, no added sugar)** – ½ cup / 125 g

Printed in Great Britain
by Amazon

56896383R00046